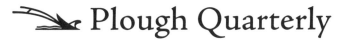

Plough Quarterly

BREAKING GROUND FOR A RENE

Summer 2018, Number 17

T0108446

Artists: Cécile Massie, Wanjin Gim, Scott Goldsmith, Michelangelo, Kyle Hartsock, Tim Lowly, Suleiman Mansour, Jan Mostaert, Erin Hanson, Zoe Cromwell

Plough Quarterly

WWW.PLOUGH.COM

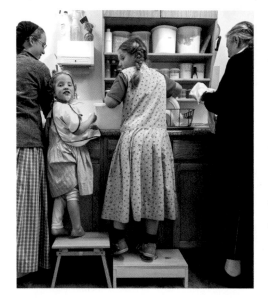

Meet the community behind *Plough*.

Plough Quarterly is published by the Bruderhof, an international community of families and singles seeking to follow Jesus together. Members of the Bruderhof are committed to a way of radical discipleship in the spirit of the Sermon on the Mount. Inspired by the first church in Jerusalem (Acts 2 and 4), they renounce private property and share everything in common in a life of nonviolence, justice, and service to neighbors near and far. The community includes people from a wide range of backgrounds. There are twenty-three Bruderhof settlements in both rural and urban locations in the United States, England, Germany, Australia, and Paraguay, with around 2,900 people in all.

To learn more or arrange a visit, see the community's website at *bruderhof.com*.

Plough Quarterly features original stories, ideas, and culture to inspire everyday faith and action. Starting from the conviction that the teachings and example of Jesus can transform and renew our world, we aim to apply them to all aspects of life, seeking common ground with all people of goodwill regardless of creed. The goal of *Plough Quarterly* is to build a living network of readers, contributors, and practitioners so that, in the words of Hebrews, we may "spur one another on toward love and good deeds."

Plough Quarterly includes contributions that we believe are worthy of our readers' consideration, whether or not we fully agree with them. Views expressed by contributors are their own and do not necessarily reflect the editorial position of *Plough* or of the Bruderhof communities.

Editors: Peter Mommsen, Veery Huleatt, Sam Hine. Art director: Emily Alexander. Managing editor: Shana Burleson.
Contributing editors: Maureen Swinger, Susannah Black.
Founding Editor: Eberhard Arnold (1883–1935).
Plough Quarterly No. 17: The Soul of Medicine
Published by Plough Publishing House, ISBN 978-0-87486-847-0
Copyright © 2018 by Plough Publishing House. All rights reserved.

Scripture quotations (unless otherwise noted) are from the New Revised Standard Version Bible, copyright © 1989 the Division of Christian Education of the National Council of the Churches of Christ in the United States of America. Used by permission. All rights reserved. Front cover image: Michelangelo, *Nude: Seated Youth and Two Studies of Arms*, c.1510/11/akgimages. Back cover artwork reproduced by permission of Zoe Cromwell.

Editorial Office	*Subscriber Services*	*United Kingdom*	*Australia*
PO Box 398	PO Box 345	Brightling Road	4188 Gwydir Highway
Walden, NY 12586	Congers, NY 10920-0345	Robertsbridge	Elsmore, NSW
T: 845.572.3455	T: 800.521.8011	TN32 5DR	2360 Australia
info@plough.com	*subscriptions@plough.com*	T: +44(0)1580.883.344	T: +61(0)2.6723.2213

Plough Quarterly (ISSN 2372-2584) is published quarterly by Plough Publishing House, PO Box 398, Walden, NY 12586.
Individual subscription $32 per year in the United States; Canada add $8, other countries add $16.
Periodicals postage paid at Walden, NY 12586 and at additional mailing offices.
POSTMASTER: Send address changes to *Plough Quarterly*, PO Box 345, Congers, NY 10920-0345.

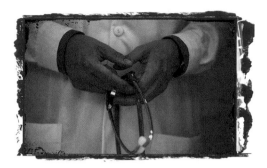

The Soul of Medicine

PETER MOMMSEN

Dear Reader,

Medicine, so long as you don't need it, is a tangential part of life, just one more profession among others. Until, that is, a loved one suffers an accident or falls sick. Then, suddenly, the doctor's findings, the lab results, and the survival statistics carry momentous importance – far more than who runs the country, who wins the World Cup, and when the polar ice caps will melt. Quite literally, it's a matter of life or death.

Medicine, of course, is also big business. US healthcare spending accounts for more than one sixth of GDP, five times more than is spent on defense. Doctors have been reclassified as "service providers," and patients are "clients" to be processed with efficiency and speed. House calls, once a routine part of practice, are now often a boutique service reserved for the rich.

Such commercialism breeds false incentives and inequalities, even in nations with healthcare systems far less profit-driven than the American one. It also has helped create tragedies like the opioid epidemic, which continues to exact a staggering toll (page 62).

Yet despite its flaws, modern medicine is in many ways a resounding humanitarian success. Over the past century, US life expectancy has leaped by thirty years. And who can argue with the elimination of smallpox and polio, or the fact that a baby born today has only one-tenth the risk of dying in infancy as one born in 1900?

Past triumphs feed expectations for medicine's future. The ability to engineer our offspring to make them smarter, more athletic, and more attractive comes nearer by the day. Will we, as the biohackers dream, figure out how to incorporate cybernetics into our bodies, gaining Superman-like powers of computation and motion? Or, as life extensionists fantasize, will we learn to reverse aging – and perhaps even seize the prize of immortality?

Freakish, yes, but there's no reason that today's fringe obsessions can't become tomorrow's mainstream causes. After all, they fit neatly into the widely held belief that medical technology will thrust constantly forward, each advance just one more step in the upward march of history. Such hopes are the beating heart of a new book by Harvard psychologist Steven Pinker, *Enlightenment Now*, in which he uses impressive statistics to argue that the world has been getting ever better since the

Enlightenment and will likely continue to do so into the future.

This optimistic story is persuasive. It's also thoroughly secular and materialist. In this way of thinking, our temporal wellbeing – the kind measured by social scientists – counts for everything, while our spiritual wellbeing counts not at all (unless it brings quantifiable benefits). God is made superfluous: according to this view, even if a supreme being does exist, he/she/it is irrelevant to securing the things that really matter – namely health, wealth, safety, and the freedom to do as we wish.

But if these are the ultimate measure of what's good for humans, it's unclear why parents shouldn't be allowed to genetically engineer elite children (page 44), or why euthanasia shouldn't be offered to anyone tired of life (page 46), or why a willing patient shouldn't be able to have his healthy legs amputated because he self-identifies as a cripple – a "treatment" that some medical ethicists actually support. In such ways, technologized medicine, which was developed to heal and sustain life, ends up warping and killing it instead.

What we need is a vision of how medicine might serve the good of the whole human person: the body's health, yes, but also the health of that "piece of divinity in us" described by the seventeenth-century physician Sir Thomas Browne. It's this divine spark that makes a child born with only part of a brain the equal in dignity and worth to a Harvard professor (page 10). It's this that explains why a life marked by ill health, poverty, danger, and constraint can still be a fulfilled one, as saints like the Beguines have shown (page 96). This is the reason why suffering, though evil in itself,

can end up being so fruitful (page 77).

We need love and reverence for humans as they are, not humans as technology may someday engineer them to be. As Pope Benedict XVI once said, "Man too has a nature that he must respect and that he cannot manipulate at will. Man is not merely self-creating freedom. Man does not create himself."

Jesus, the healer from Nazareth, showed what it means to love the imperfect, the frail, the average, those whom no one would mistake for a designer baby. He commanded his followers to care in practical ways for "the least of these my brethren," whether by comforting the sick or offering the hungry food and the thirsty drink.

The glory of the medical profession is that it is dedicated to these works of mercy. In today's money-driven healthcare industry, such tasks are often poorly rewarded. Yet they're at the heart of medicine's original mission.

My mother, a family doctor, often used to point out the power of small actions in caring for a person: adjusting a pillow, clearing away a tray, making a joke on the way out. (An interview with her and her colleague is on page 17.) Such little things don't eliminate pain or abolish dying. But they have lasting value: they are foretastes of the day promised in the Book of Revelation, when God "will wipe away every tear from their eyes, and death shall be no more." These are the things that make up the soul of medicine.

Warm greetings,

Peter Mommsen
Editor

> # We need love and reverence for humans as they are.

Beloved Community

On Peter Mommsen's "The Prophet We Need Now," Spring 2018: Peter Mommsen implies Josiah Royce had no respect for Christ, and that seemed a bit unfair to me.

Royce (1855–1916) was an American philosopher who was concerned with questions of religion and the philosophy of community. Although he never joined a church, Royce was deeply familiar with scripture and understood that humankind needed to be saved from its fallen nature.

In fact, he had great respect for the early Christian communities and their foundation on Christ's teachings, as vividly described in Paul's epistles. "To Paul's mind," Royce wrote, "[Christ's] mission was divine. He both knew and loved his community before it existed on earth; for his foreknowledge was one with that of the God whose will he came to accomplish. On earth he called into this community its first members. He suffered and died that it might have life. Through his death and in his life the community lives. He is now identical with the spirit of this community."

Royce considered these consciously cooperative communities to be full of grace, and in pondering their meaning he came to think of them as a prime example of what he called the "beloved community." He later developed this concept in his book, *The Problem of Christianity,* which was to influence Martin Luther King Jr.'s vision of the beloved community as the goal of the civil rights movement.

George Albertz, Rifton, NY

Who Is My Neighbor?

On D. L. Mayfield's "For the Love of Neighbor," Spring 2018: I'm a member of a small, rural, mostly white church in the South. I wanted to share a really encouraging moment that happened a week ago in a committee meeting

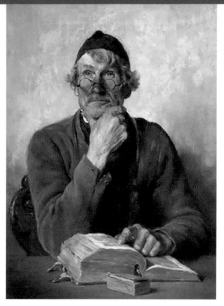

Hugo Kauffmann, *Elderly Reader*

at church. I told my husband I wanted to send D. L. Mayfield's article to this committee to start a conversation, but he wasn't hopeful. "It won't do any good," he said. "You'll just make people mad." Well, I sent it anyway.

What a surprise at our next committee meeting when the woman leading our devotional read the Good Samaritan story out of Luke. She then said, "I am so glad I read that article. It is really challenging me. As one of those people who has supported building a wall and limiting Muslim immigration, I had never considered that my neighbor might be someone who lived outside of the United States. I'm rethinking everything now."

I was floored! And excited. We had a really good conversation after she opened up the conversation in such a vulnerable way. Minds can change and challenging conversations can happen! *Grace (location withheld)*

We welcome letters to the editor. Letters and web comments may be edited for length and clarity, and may be published in any medium. Letters should be sent with the writer's name and address to letters@plough.com.

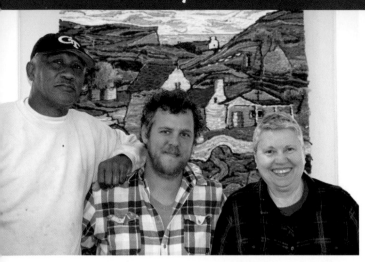

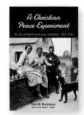

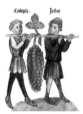

Koinonia Farm residents, *from left,* Norris Harris, Steve Krout, and Bren Dubay offered history and comments at the 75th anniversary.

Photograph by Cindi Cox, *Albany Herald.* Used with permission.

Celebrating 75 Years at Koinonia Farm

Although it's been almost fifty years since Clarence Jordan died in a tiny shack in rural Georgia, his influence has continued to spread and grow, as demonstrated by the diverse crowd – octogenarian locals, young activists, seasoned communitarians, and farming enthusiasts – that turned out to celebrate his legacy this spring. A farmer and Southern Baptist preacher, Jordan founded Koinonia Farm in 1942 as a "demonstration plot for the kingdom," a place where he and others could live out economic and racial justice in community. In spite of a hostile local reception, including KKK violence and a boycott, the community has survived to this day. In a remarkable change of heart, two local churches that fifty years ago had expelled the Koinonia members for bringing a black man into the sanctuary vied for the honor of hosting the conference. *koinoniafarm.org*

Theology of the People of God

"Theology of the People of God," a new distance learning program at the Pontifical Lateran University in Rome, offers a two-year course of study in English and German. Cardinal Kurt Koch, President of the Pontifical Council for Promoting Christian Unity, said of the correspondence course: "Drawing on the theme of God's people, this theology brings together the various theological disciplines into one whole, which comes from the root of Israel. The questions of faith and Church posed by modern man in the time after the Enlightenment must be taken up consistently." The topics examined during the course include: "Why Christianity isn't a 'religion,'" "Why Judaism is indispensible to the Church," and "How faith and history are connected."

"Theology of the People of God" is a project of the Catholic Integrated Community (CIC), which was founded in Germany in the aftermath of World War II and the Holocaust. Led by Herbert and Traudl Wallbrecher, young people gathered to ask why the Christians of their time had failed to oppose the Nazi regime's ideology and atrocities. Now with a membership that includes laity and priests, families and singles, the CIC seeks to be a place where "people can live the fullness of Christianity with a modern approach to faith and reason."

Find out more about the new theology program at *popolodidio.org/en/distance-learning.*

Bruderhof in Britain

In *A Christian Peace Experiment: The Bruderhof Community in Britain, 1933–1942* (Cascade, 2018), Professor Ian M. Randall meticulously researches and narrates a fascinating and somewhat forgotten chapter in the history of the Bruderhof movement. From the back cover:

> After the rise to power of the Nazi regime, the Bruderhof became a target and the

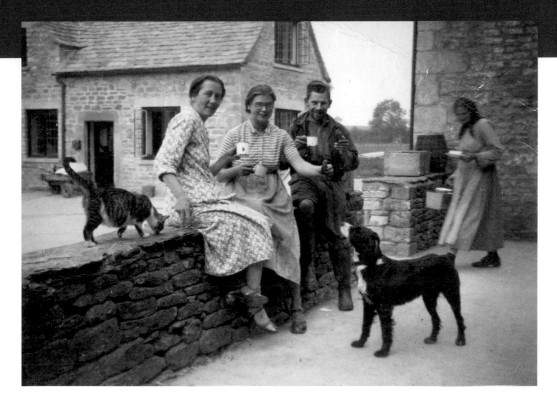

community was forcibly dissolved. Members who escaped from Germany and traveled to England were welcomed as refugees from persecution and a community was established in the Cotswolds.

In the period from 1933 to 1942, when the Bruderhof's witness was advancing in Britain, its members were in touch with many individuals and movements. This book covers the Bruderhof's connections with (among others) the Fellowship of Reconciliation, Dietrich Bonhoeffer, the Peace Pledge Union, the social work of Muriel and Doris Lester in East London, Jewish refugee groups, and artistic pioneers like Eric Gill. As significant numbers of British people joined the Bruderhof, its farming, publishing, and arts and crafts activities extended considerably. But with the outbreak of the Second World War, German members came to be regarded with suspicion and British members became unpopular locally because they were pacifists.

Although the Bruderhof was defended in Parliament, notably by Lady Astor, it seemed that German members would be interned as enemy aliens. The consequence was that by 1942 over three hundred community members had left England. With Mennonite assistance, they began to forge a new life in South America. This book traces a remarkable Christian peace experiment being undertaken in a time of great political upheaval.

Readers can expect an intriguing glimpse into community life, pre–Second World War Britain, and the very first issue of *Plough!*

Poet in This Issue: Suzanne Harlan Heyd

Heyd, whose poems appear on pages 61 and 69, lives with her seminary professor husband in Manila, Philippines. She has lived in Egypt, Jordan, Sudan, Lebanon, and Iraq, and hopes to live again in the Arabic-speaking world. She has an MFA in creative writing from Seattle Pacific University and a forthcoming EP, "Remember Me," with a handful of songs for the Middle East. ➣

Tea break at the Cotswold Bruderhof, England, 1940. Winifred Pacey, *second from left*, then an Oxford philosophy student, later became a *Plough* editor.

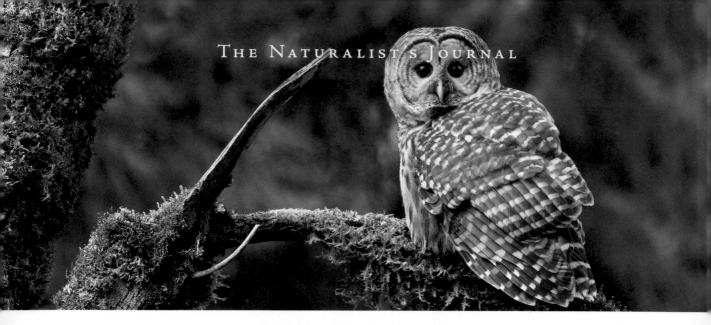

The Hunter

DWIGHT WAREHAM

EARLY ON SUNDAY MORNING two friends and I hiked along the Wallkill River, hoping to see white-tailed deer. We were walking along a dirt lane bordered with a sixty-foot strip of open meadow and then forest on the left with a deciduous woods on the right. Our eyes were up looking for deer when we noticed a gray oval shape on a tree branch in a low solitary tree ahead to the left. The binoculars came out and to our amazement we saw that it was a barred owl. We immediately gave up on deer and began stalking this owl, getting closer and closer until we were within fifty-five feet of it. It was perched about twelve feet off the ground and although the sun had not risen yet, daylight was advancing.

We stood motionless for half an hour and watched it hunting for its breakfast. Twice it leaped from its perch and pounced into the grass, probably after a meadow vole, which we were unable to see. Both times it returned to its perch and gazed downwards with its dark brown eyes. Occasionally migrating birds would pass high overhead and it would crane its neck back and watch them fly by before returning its gaze to the action below.

After some minutes, the owl was spotted by a white-breasted nuthatch passing by. The smaller bird immediately started scolding and before long the warning "jay, jay" of an approaching blue jay was heard. I could hear reinforcements coming from the distance. Soon a mob of blue jays and nuthatches was attacking the owl. The owl quickly had enough and glided away into the forest on absolutely silent wings. The jays and nuthatches were mystified as to where it had gone and started systematically searching the branches of the tree where it had been, without success. Eventually they dispersed.

Now the owl leaped from its sheltered perch. Coming straight toward us with wings straight out to the sides, it returned to a nearby tree to resume its hunting. ⤳

Dwight Wareham is an avid naturalist and a veteran elementary school teacher. He lives at the Mount Community, a Bruderhof in Esopus, New York.

Photograph by Stiles Williams

Beyond Racial Reconciliation

JOHN M. PERKINS

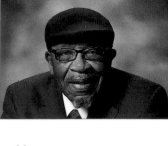

I'VE GIVEN MOST of my life to the cause of reconciliation, fighting the battle in the trenches and working with community development organizations. We developed the three Rs – relocation, reconciliation, and redistribution – to offer a process to help communities work together to balance some of the inequities of life in America. By God's grace, much good work has been done, and I'm humbled to have been a part of it.

But as I come closer to the end of my journey, I am aware that community development can only take us so far – because this is a gospel issue. The problem of reconciliation in our country and in our churches is much too big to be wrestled to the ground by plans that begin in the minds of men. This is a God-sized problem. It is one that only the church, through the power of the Holy Spirit, can heal. It requires the quality of love that only our Savior can provide. And it requires that we make some uncomfortable confessions. G. K. Chesterton said, "It isn't that they can't see the solution. It is that they can't see the problem." I believe this statement can be applied to the lack of reconciliation within the church today.

The problem is that there is a gaping hole in our gospel. We have preached a gospel that leaves us believing that we can be reconciled to God but not reconciled to our Christian brothers and sisters who don't look like us – brothers and sisters with whom we are, in fact, one blood.

The apostle John talks about that: "If someone says, 'I love God,' and hates his brother, he is a liar; for the one who does not love his brother whom he has seen, cannot love God whom he has not seen" (1 John 4:20). Yet from our early days as a country we adopted the practice of slavery and demonized the slave as inferior, subhuman, and deserving of exploitation. For this wicked system of slavery to survive there had to be distinctions made between normal folks and this new breed of people that would be treated like animals. This is where the idea of race came into play.

The truth is that there is no black race – and there is no white race. So the idea of "racial reconciliation" is a false idea. It's a lie. It implies that there is more than one race. This is absolutely false. God created only one race – the human race.

We're at a unique moment in our history. We've come through – and in many ways are in the midst of – great upheaval. The soul of our nation has been laid bare. We have only to look at the signs of the times to realize that the church may not have long to get this right. We may not have much time left to offer the world a glimpse of this unity that will point the eyes of the watching world to the power of our great God. Yes, there's an urgency. Time is running out . . . for all of us. But while we still have time, let's reflect on the heart of Jesus, who prayed that his church might one day be one. ⟵

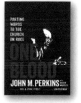

Dr. John M. Perkins, born in 1930 to Mississippi sharecroppers, is a pastor, author, and civil rights activist. This article is taken from his new book, One Blood: Parting Words to the Church on Race, *with Karen Waddles (Moody, 2018). Used by permission.*

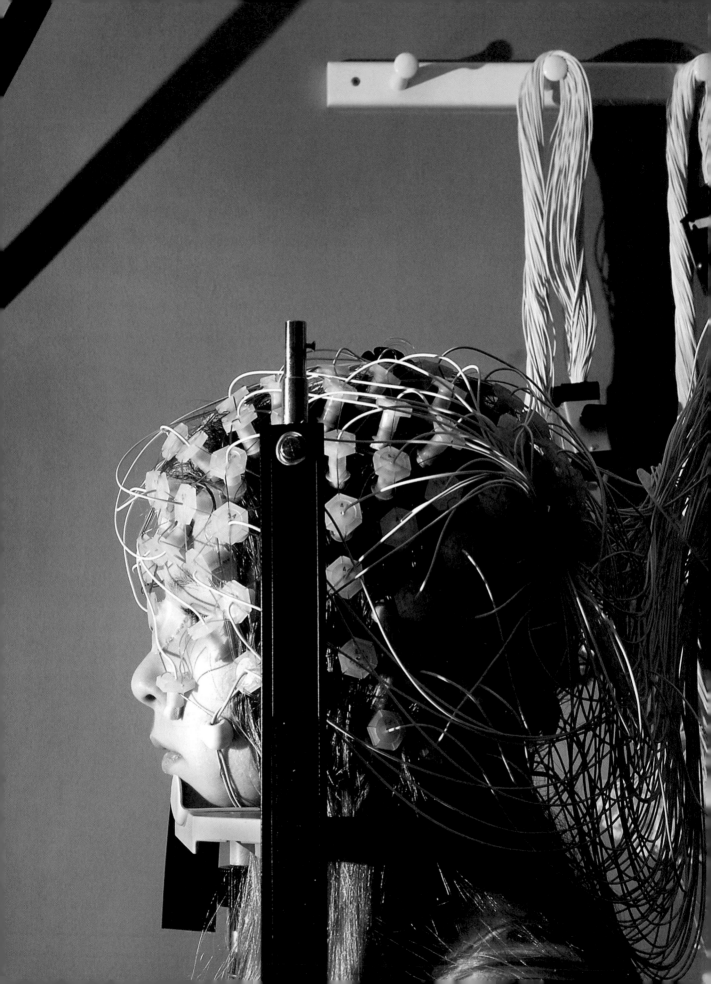

The
Science
of the
Soul

MICHAEL EGNOR

Previous spread: A twelve-year-old participates in brain research at the University of Pittsburgh Medical Center. Photograph by Scott Goldsmith.

I watched the CAT scan images appear on the screen, one by one. The baby's head was mostly empty. There were only thin slivers of brain – a bit of brain tissue at the base of the skull, and a thin rim around the edges. The rest was water.

Her parents had feared this. We had seen it on the prenatal ultrasound; the CAT scan, hours after birth, was much more accurate. Katie looked like a normal newborn, but she had little chance at a normal life. She had a fraternal-twin sister in the incubator next to her. But Katie only had a third of the brain that her sister had. I explained all of this to her family, trying to keep alive a flicker of hope for their daughter.

I cared for Katie as she grew up. At every stage of Katie's life so far, she has excelled. She sat and talked and walked earlier than her sister. She's made the honor roll. She will soon graduate high school.

I've had other patients whose brains fell far short of their minds. Maria had only two-thirds of a brain. She needed a couple of operations to drain fluid, but she thrives. She just finished her master's degree in English literature, and is a published musician. Jesse was born with a head shaped like a football and half-full of water – doctors told his mother to let him die at birth. She disobeyed. He is a normal happy middle-schooler, loves sports, and wears his hair long.

Some people with deficient brains are profoundly handicapped. But not all are. I've treated and cared for scores of kids who grow up with brains that are deficient but minds that thrive. How is this possible? Neuroscience, and Thomas Aquinas, point to the answer.

Is the Mind Mechanical?

As a medical student, I fell in love with the brain. It's a daunting organ: an ensemble of cells and axons and nuclei and lobes tucked and folded in exotic shapes. I had to learn what it looks like when it's sliced through by CAT scans, and then what it looks like when I slice through it. My fascination with neuroanatomy was metaphysical: this was where our thoughts and decisions came from, this was a roadmap of the human self, and I was learning to read it as I read a book. It was the truth about us, I thought.

But I was wrong. Katie made me face my misunderstanding. She was a whole person. The child in my office was not mapped in any meaningful way to the scan of her brain or the diagram in my neuroanatomy textbook. The roadmap got it wrong.

How does the mind relate to the brain? This question is central to my professional life. I thought I had it answered. Yet a century of research and thirty years of my own neurosurgical practice have challenged everything I thought I knew.

Michael Egnor, MD, is a neurosurgeon and professor of neurological surgery and pediatrics at Stony Brook University.

The view assumed by those who taught me is that the mind is wholly a product of the brain, which is itself understood as something like a machine. Francis Crick, a neuroscientist and the Nobel laureate who was the co-discoverer of the structure of DNA, wrote that "a person's mental activities are entirely due to the behavior of nerve cells, glial cells, and the atoms, ions, and molecules that make them up and influence them."

This mechanical philosophy is the result of two steps. It began with Rene Descartes, who argued that the mind and the brain were separate substances, immaterial and material. Somehow (how, neither Descartes nor anyone else can say) the mind is linked to the brain – it's the ghost in the machine.

But as Francis Bacon's approach to understanding the world gained ascendency during the scientific Enlightenment, it became fashionable to limit inquiry about the world to physical substances: to study the machine and ignore the ghost. Matter was tractable, and we studied it to obsession. The ghost was ignored, and then denied. This was what the logic of materialism demanded.

The materialist insists that we are slaves of our neurons, without genuine free will. Materialism comes in different flavors, each having passed into and then out of favor over the past century, as their insufficiency became apparent. Behaviorists asserted that the mind, if it exists at all, is irrelevant. All that matters is what is observable – input and output. Yet behaviorism is in eclipse, because it's difficult to deny the relevance of the mind to neuroscience.

> # The brain can be cut in half, but the intellect and will cannot.

Identity theory, replacing behaviorism, held that the mind just is the brain. Thoughts and sensations are exactly the same thing as brain tissue and neurotransmitters, understood differently. The pain you feel in your finger is identical to the nerve impulses in your arm and in your brain. But, of course, that's not really true. Pain hurts and nerve impulses are electrical and chemical. They're not even similar. Identity theorists struggled with uncooperative reality for a generation, then gave up.

Computer functionalism came next: the brain is hardware and mind is software. But this too has problems. Nineteenth-century German philosopher Franz Brentano pointed out that the one thing that absolutely distinguishes thoughts from matter is that thoughts are always *about* something, and matter is never *about* anything. This aboutness is the hallmark of the mind. Every thought has a meaning. No material thing has meaning.

Computation is the mapping of an input to an output according to an algorithm, irrespective of meaning. Computation has no aboutness; it is the antithesis of thought.

Neuroscience and Metaphysics

Remarkably, neuroscience tells us three things about the mind: the mind is metaphysically simple, the intellect and will are immaterial, and free will is real.

In the middle of the twentieth century, neurosurgeons discovered that they could treat a certain kind of epilepsy by severing a large bundle of brain fibers, called the corpus callosum, which connects the two hemispheres of the brain. Following these operations, each hemisphere worked independently. But what happened to the mind of a person with his or her brain split in half?

The neuroscientist Roger Sperry studied scores of split-brain patients. He found, surprisingly, that in ordinary life the patients showed little effect. Each patient was still one person. The intellect and will – the capacity to have abstract thought and to choose – remained unified. Only by meticulous testing could Sperry find any differences: their *perceptions* were altered by the surgery. Sensations – elicited by touch or vision – could be presented to one hemisphere of the brain, and not be experienced in the other hemisphere. Speech production is associated with the left hemisphere of the brain; patients could not name an object presented to the right hemisphere (via the left visual field). Yet they could point to the object with their left hand (which is controlled by the right hemisphere). The most remarkable result of Sperry's Nobel Prize–winning work was that the person's intellect and will – what we might call the soul – remained undivided.

The brain can be cut in half, but the intellect and will cannot. The intellect and will are metaphysically simple.

One of the neurosurgeons who pioneered the corpus callosotomy for epilepsy patients was Wilder Penfield, who worked in Montreal in the middle of the twentieth century. Penfield studied the brains and minds of epileptic patients in a remarkably direct way, in the course of treating them. He operated on people who were awake. The brain itself feels no pain, and local anesthetics numb the scalp and skull enough to permit painless brain surgery. Penfield asked them to do and think things while he was observing and temporarily stimulating or impairing regions of their brains. Two things astonished him.

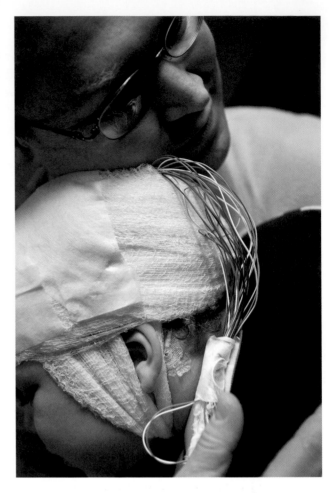

First, he noticed something about seizures. He could cause seizures by stimulating the brain. A patient would jerk his arm, or feel tingling, or see flashes of light, or even have memories. But what he could never do was cause an *intellectual* seizure: the patient would never reason when his brain was stimulated. The patient never contemplated mercy or bemoaned injustice or calculated second derivatives in response to brain stimulation. If the brain wholly gives rise to the mind, why are there no intellectual seizures?

Second, Penfield noted that patients always knew that the movement or sensation elicited by brain stimulation was done *to* them, but not *by* them. When Penfield stimulated the arm area of the brain, patients always said, "You made my arm move" and never said, "I moved my arm." Patients always retained a correct awareness of agency. There was a part of the patient – the will – that Penfield could not reach with his electrode.

Penfield began his career as a materialist. He finished his career as an emphatic dualist. He insisted that there is an aspect of the self – the intellect and the will – that is not the brain, and that cannot be elicited by stimulation of the brain.

Some of the most fascinating research on consciousness was done by Penfield's contemporary Benjamin Libet at the University of California, San Francisco. Libet asked: What happens in the brain when we think? How are electrical signals in the brain related to our thoughts? He was particularly interested in the timing of brain waves and thoughts. Did a brain wave happen at the same moment as the thought, or before, or after?

It was a difficult question to answer. It wasn't hard to measure electrical changes in the brain: that could be done routinely by electrodes on the scalp, and Libet enlisted neurosurgeons to allow him to record signals deep in the brain while patients were awake. The challenge Libet faced was to accurately measure the time interval between the signals and the thoughts. But the signals last only a few milliseconds, and how can you time a thought with that kind of accuracy?

Libet began by choosing a very simple thought: the decision to press a button. He modified an oscilloscope so that a dot circled the screen once each second, and when the subject decided to push the button, he or she noted the location of the dot at the time of the decision. Libet measured the timing of the decision and the timing of the brain waves of

We are composites of matter and spirit.

many volunteers with accuracy in the tens of milliseconds. Consistently he found that the conscious decision to push the button was preceded by about half a second by a brain wave, which he called the readiness potential.

Then a half-second later the subject became aware of his decision. It appeared at first that the subjects were not free; their brains made the decision to move and they followed it.

But Libet looked deeper. He asked his subjects to veto their decision immediately after they made it – to not push the button. Again, the readiness potential appeared a half-second before conscious awareness of the decision to push the button, but Libet found that the veto – he called it "free won't" – had no brain wave corresponding to it.

The brain, then, has activity that corresponds to a pre-conscious urge to do something. But we are free to veto or accept this urge. The motives are material. The veto, and implicitly the acceptance, is an immaterial act of the will.

Libet noted the correspondence between his experiments and the traditional religious understanding of human beings. We are, he said, beset by a sea of inclinations, corresponding to material activity in our brains, which we have the free choice to reject or accept. It is hard not to read this in more familiar terms: we are tempted by sin, yet we are free to choose.

The approach to understanding the world and ourselves that was replaced by materialism was that of classical metaphysics. This tradition's most notable investigator and teacher was Saint Thomas Aquinas. Following Aristotle, Aquinas wrote that the human soul has distinct kinds of abilities. Vegetative powers, shared by plants and animals, serve growth, nourishment, and metabolism. Sensitive powers, shared with animals, include perception, passions, and locomotion. The vegetative and sensitive powers are material abilities of the brain.

Yet human beings have two powers of the soul that are not material – intellect and will. These transcend matter. They are the means by which we reason, and by which we choose based on reason. We are composites of matter and spirit. We have spiritual souls.

Aquinas would not be surprised by the results of these researchers' investigations.

What's at Stake

Philosopher Roger Scruton has written that contemporary neuroscience is "a vast collection of answers with no memory of the questions." Materialism has limited the kinds of questions that we're allowed to ask, but neuroscience, pursued without a materialist bias, points towards the reality that we are chimeras: material beings with immaterial souls.

How would our lives or our society be different if we found that our mind was merely the product of our material brain – and that our every decision was determined, with no free will?

The cornerstone of totalitarianism, according to Hannah Arendt, is the denial of free will. Under the visions of Communism and Nazism, we are mere instruments of historical forces, not individual free agents who can choose good or evil.

Without free will, we cannot be guilty in an individual sense. But we also cannot be innocent. Neither the Jews under Hitler nor Kulak farmers under Stalin were killed because they were individually at fault. Their guilt was assigned to them according to their type, and accordingly they were exterminated to hasten a natural process, whether the purification of the race or the dictatorship of the proletariat.

By contrast, the classical understanding of human nature is that we are free beings not subject to determinism. This understanding is the indispensable basis for human liberty and dignity. It is indispensable, too, for simply making sense of the world around us: among other things, for making sense of Katie.

I see her in my office each year. She is thriving: headstrong and bright. Her mother is exasperated, and, after seventeen years, still surprised. So am I.

There is much about the brain and the mind that I don't understand. But neuroscience tells a consistent story. There is a part of Katie's mind that is not her brain. She is more than that. She can reason and she can choose. There is a part of her that is immaterial – the part that Sperry couldn't split, that Penfield couldn't reach, and that Libet couldn't find with his electrodes. There is a part of Katie that didn't show up on those CAT scans when she was born.

Katie, like you and me, has a soul. ⤴

Recommended Reading

The Philosophy of Mind: A Short Introduction
Edward Feser (Oneworld, 2005)

Aquinas: A Beginner's Guide
Edward Feser (Oneworld, 2009)

Mind Time: The Temporal Factor in Consciousness
Benjamin Libet (Harvard, 2005)

Mystery of the Mind: A Critical Study of Consciousness and the Human Brain
Wilder Penfield (Princeton, 2015)

The Origins of Totalitarianism
Hannah Arendt (Andesite, 2017)

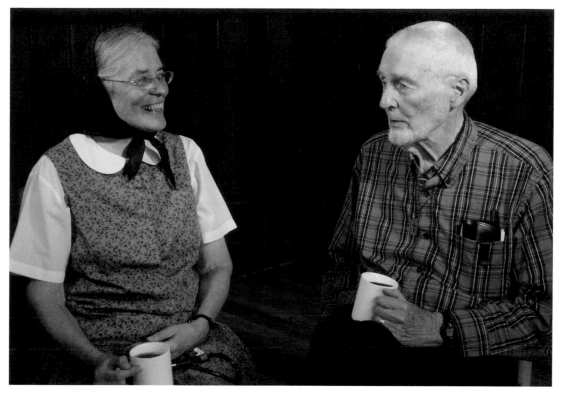

Monika Mommsen and Milton Zimmerman

Money-Free
Medicine

MONIKA MOMMSEN AND MILTON ZIMMERMAN

What's it like to practice medicine in a community where doctors don't
charge and patients don't pay? *Plough* sat down with two Bruderhof
physicians to talk about house calls, new technologies, the moments
of birth and death – and why having fun is a vital part of care.

Plough: *How did you get into medicine?*

Milton Zimmerman: When I was four years old I had rheumatic fever. The doctor who took care of me came on house calls again and again, and he was such a friendly guy whom I enjoyed so much. I thought, "Hey, when I grow up I want to be like him." That's where it started. After Amherst, I attended the University of Pennsylvania Medical School, class of '54.

> **"One of the most special experiences is to see a new soul arrive in the world and hear that first cry."**
>
> *Monika Mommsen*

During medical school I found Jesus – or Jesus found me. That set a direction for my life, and I was looking for a church that really followed the Sermon on the Mount and Jesus' life and teachings. That led me to become a pacifist. As a result, in 1957, when I was looking for a place to do my alternative service in lieu of going to the military, I chose the Bruderhof-run hospital in Paraguay. Two years later, my wife and I joined the community.

I practiced medicine for sixty years. All but two of those were as a family doctor working within the Bruderhof community – mostly treating community members, but also working at the local hospital and in the clinic treating migrant farmers nearby.

Monika Mommsen: I've practiced for forty-one years. Ever since I was little, I had always wanted to be a nurse – I grew up in the Bruderhof community. But in my senior year of high school, after I expressed my wish to become a member, the community asked if I would become a doctor, since they were eager to have a female physician. That came as a surprise, but I said yes and I've loved it ever since. After getting an undergraduate art degree I studied at the Albany Medical College, class of '75. From the beginning, Milton has been my mentor.

Plough: *Were there other women doctors in the Bruderhof community at the time?*

Monika: Yes, two English women doctors had joined in England before World War II and moved down to Paraguay, South America, where they helped found a hospital. But they weren't practicing much anymore. And Dr. Miriam Brailey, a pioneering epidemiologist who had taught at the Johns Hopkins School of Medicine, was also a Bruderhof member and a family friend.

Medicine in Community

Plough: *Practicing in a Christian community like the Bruderhof, you are able to offer cradle-to-grave care. What does this look like?*

Milton: Well, our care is better than cradle-to-grave – it starts six months before the cradle. Isn't that right, Monika?

Monika: Often mothers confide in me if they think they may be pregnant. We usually see them in the office at twelve weeks when we can hear the heartbeat. Of course, we offer them best-practice prenatal care, and if there is any cause for concern, we'll make sure a mother is seen by a qualified specialist. But one of the most wonderful things I can tell them is that actually there is so little doctors can do medically at this stage other than monitor – God is in control of this pregnancy. In a way, the fact that medicine's ability to intervene is

---

Milton Zimmerman, MD, and Monika Mommsen, MD, live at Woodcrest, a Bruderhof in Rifton, New York.

so limited before the birth can be a healthy reminder to focus on what's most important: that here we are witnessing a mystery, the creation of a new life.

I'm usually present at the birth, which takes place very much in the context of prayer – and joy. That is one of the most special experiences, to see a new soul arrive in the world and hear that first cry, which is vital for the little one's life really – to take that first deep breath of air, to cry.

Then I'm there for all the checkups and immunizations, and there may be the normal childhood events like bronchiolitis and ear infections, and later, teenage acne. Then I see them again when they get married and start having children. Recently, I've begun to see the grandchildren of people I first cared for as children.

Plough: *Do you use alternative therapies?*

Monika: No, it's conventional, science-based medicine.

Plough: *As physicians, you are also the ones present when people face a tragedy.*

Monika: There are very hard moments – for example, accompanying a mother through a birth when she knows that the child is not alive. Yet it can be a very moving experience to welcome a child who was already taken, realizing that this child had very much value in God's eyes and had already done its work on earth, even while inside the mother. Then it's our privilege to grieve with the parents and do what we can so this is an experience their family, and the community, can share with them.

Every child, even an early miscarriage, has a message – certainly for the father and mother, but also for everyone who is involved. One's reverence for life, for the preciousness of life, only grows as you get older, I think.

Plough: *Outside of a communal way of life, medicine is typically practiced in a commercial environment: money flows between doctor and patient, between doctor and his or her employer, and from both doctor and patient to their insurance companies. What difference does it make to practice medicine without it being a monetary transaction?*

PATIENT PERSPECTIVE

DORLI ALBERTZ

As told to Erna Albertz

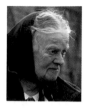

When I was diagnosed with terminal cancer two years ago, I didn't know what it would mean, but one thing I did know was that I wouldn't have to worry about how I would be cared for. My doctor is Monika Mommsen, who is a fellow member of the Bruderhof community here.

When I was first diagnosed I would make the five-minute walk to her office in the Bruderhof clinic for my appointments, but now that I don't get around as easily she has started visiting me at home. Our visits are informal – she asks about my work (I translate documents saved from the Bruderhof's beginnings from German to English) and we swap stories about our grandchildren.

Dorli Albertz, age eighty-four, is a former kindergarten teacher who lives in upstate New York.

Milton: When I first started practicing medicine, I had my own family practice in a semi-rural area outside Philadelphia. I charged $3.50 for an office visit and $5.00 for a house call. Can you imagine? But I was able to pay off my debts within one year and it was a lot of fun. You can't get around it, though: the monetary transaction between doctor and patient is always there in the background defining the relationship.

Here in the Bruderhof, it's not there at all. Because we share a common purse, money is irrelevant to both the patient and me, and has no bearing on the care we give. That allows a relationship of full trust between doctor and patient to a degree that's rarely possible elsewhere.

Monika: It frees us to care for somebody as a human being first and foremost. We get no pay, so whatever I do or don't do doesn't affect my income. In conventional medicine nowadays, doctors have to see twenty to twenty-five patients in a day, every ten to fifteen minutes, and there's just no time that they can actually take to listen. Here we have that time and we're not driven by economics. Also, the relationship between colleagues (there are about a dozen Bruderhof doctors), nurses, and staff is close because we have the same faith and are committed to this community. There are no employer-employee relationships between us.

Still, my practice is not just for community members. I also have patients from our neighborhood who don't have money, and I always do it for free. I have such joy in doing that – it actually makes it easier to care for someone if there isn't an economic reward system involved.

Plough: *So this gives you the freedom to make house calls?*

Monika: Absolutely. For example, I will often visit a mother at home with her new baby. You get an entirely different impression of both of them, and you have a cup of tea together and talk about how things like feeding are going – it's much less formal. I'll do the same

Patient Perspective, *continued*

It's usually only incidentally that we touch on any bothersome symptoms. That doesn't mean she forgets her job: as soon as she identifies a medical issue, she is immediately attentive to it and focused on finding a solution. She has explained the treatment options to me but respects my wish to continue to live fully – and be kept comfortable and functioning as much as possible – but to refrain from unnecessary tests or procedures.

Of course, my illness affects my day-to-day life, and in community it is possible for Monika to work with other community members who can help make changes to my living environment. For example, when I began to need a hospital bed, but our bedroom was too small for one, she simply contacted the person responsible for housing here at our Woodcrest community to set in motion a plan to relocate us – George, my husband of forty-one years, our daughter Erna, and me – to a larger apartment. Additional perks of our new quarters include a walk-in shower and spare room to store pieces of medical equipment such as a wheelchair and walker. When moving day came, two or three neighbors were on hand to help with all the heavy lifting and with setting up the bed. By the end of the day, a woman who works in our community laundry had arrived with linens to fit my new mattress. If the time comes when I need more if a mother has a sick child on the weekend, and certainly for patients who are getting older – after a certain point, I basically do not see them in the office at all – it's just home visits. Of course, everything's much more convenient in the office, but I think it shows care to come to someone's home.

Milton: You also learn a lot about what's going on – to see how the family interacts with the patient, whether the neighbors are supportive, whether the house is messy or too scrupulously clean.

Monika: If a patient needs to go to the emergency room or visit a specialist, we'll often go with them. In these situations, our job is to be our patients' advocates. Often the specialists are very surprised that the patient is bringing her own personal doctor, but generally they're appreciative, and we certainly get much better care that way.

Technology and Medicine

Plough: Over the decades that you've been practicing, researchers have developed increasingly powerful forms of technology, from fertility treatments to experimental cancer drugs to life support that can keep people alive for years. What are your views on the technologization of medicine?

Milton: Rightly used, many of the new technologies can be a tremendous blessing. But so often technology is put at the service of money, not of the patient's best interests. Medicine used to be a profession, but it has turned into a business – so openly, so blatantly. Mammon drives the so-called healthcare industry from top to bottom. (I won't even talk about the pharmaceutical companies.) So the doctors end up ordering too many tests and treatments that don't actually benefit patients. Insurance covers big operations and expensive drugs, but not the day-to-day care that would, for example, be of far more value to an elderly person than a dramatic intervention.

A related factor in the use of technology is doctors' strong drive to overcome a disease – to "win the battle" by curing the patient. Again, in its right place this drive can help motivate

nursing care, that will be provided as well, right here in our apartment, where my grandchildren and the neighbors' children run in and out and their parents stop through to collect them or have a cup of tea while they play. For the moment, my wheelchair enables me to go out of our house several times a day, to spend time with other women in the community laundry folding clothes for families, to go to daily community gatherings, or just to enjoy being out-of-doors.

I also require a special diet; here again, Monika let the community kitchen team know, and it is a matter of course for them to provide me with the food I need. It is probably hard for someone who

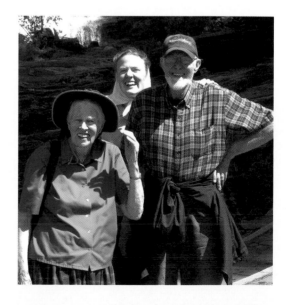

With my husband, George, and daughter Erna

us to do our very best to help someone. But it also can influence the doctor's decision-making in a harmful way, where "winning" becomes more important than caring for the patient. For example, three years ago my daughter-in-law was dying of cancer. On her last visit to one oncologist, she was abruptly and curtly dismissed with the words, "I have nothing more to offer you." The oncologist recognized that he could no longer "win," and as a result ceased caring for the patient. She and her husband walked out feeling crushed.

But there's *always* more we can do for a patient. I learned that early on after I started practicing in the community, when a mother brought in a child with a high fever. I checked him over – everything was OK; it was just a viral infection that would run its course, and the boy was in no danger. I said to the mother, "He doesn't need antibiotics; there's nothing more to do here."

She put her hands on her hips and looked at me with a real scowl and said, "Is that all they taught you in medical school? What this child needs is aspirin, juice, and love. Don't tell me there's nothing more to do!" And she was right – we can't always offer a cure, but we can always offer care.

Monika: Technology can give us the illusion that we're in control. Yet as human beings, we have to accept that not everything is how we wish. For example, I'm all for helping a woman who has problems conceiving, but there comes a limit. How can it be right to use in vitro fertilization if it results in so many frozen unwanted embryos? Obviously, there are countless forms of medical technology that I am grateful for. But there is a time to step back.

A technology-focused approach to medicine also interferes with the doctor–patient relationship. I recently visited an eye doctor, and apart from glancing at me maybe twice, she spent

> ## "There's absolutely no conflict between asking God for healing while also using medicine."
>
> *Milton Zimmerman*

PATIENT PERSPECTIVE, *continued*

hasn't experienced it to imagine how completely someone can be cared for in a community. But it goes beyond practicalities. One of our pastors, Milton Zimmerman (who is also a retired doctor) and his wife, Sandy, often spend time with George and me to find out how we are doing. We can share any worries that have arisen – or anything that has recently inspired us – and receive their guidance. And at a communal meal, I may end up sitting right across the table from Monika, or Milton, or the diet cook, or one of the people who helped set up my bed – and converse with them simply as a fellow pilgrim on this path of committed community. This is just everyday living

for me, but I hope I never forget that it is radical everyday living.

Another thing I do not have to worry about is the care of my youngest daughter, Iris, who has Down syndrome. Because Erna is caring for me and my other daughter, Ria, has young children, neither is able to look after Iris at the moment. So a young woman has moved in next to her to be a companion to her. It is a great gift to be able to face the end of my days on earth knowing that Iris is in good hands.

Before we moved apartments, we lived next door to Ria, her husband Norman, and their four little ones, and I watched as they too received the her whole time on the computer. We're losing the priceless value of examining, of touching a patient.

Milton: This subject was covered in a recent *New York Times Magazine* article by Dr. Abraham Verghese, professor of internal medicine at Stanford University, who described his own experience as a hospital patient. Too often the doctors and nurses were totally engrossed in the monitors and lab reports and imaging. He comments, "I received care but did not feel cared for."

Monika: Even at the end of life when there's actually nothing you can do because they're dying – if they have pain, touch them, examine them. I learned the importance of this from my sister, who died a few years ago of metastatic cancer. When I examined her, she felt that I heard her and was listening to her, that I was legitimizing her worry. I would be honest and say, "Yes, the mass is growing."

Medicine and Faith

Plough: *Some Christians seem to feel there is a contradiction between trusting in medicine and believing in prayer. Do you see that as a conflict?*

Monika: Not at all. I think it always has to go together. I often pray before I see someone, especially in situations where I don't know what to do or am having difficulty, so that my frustration doesn't show in my encounter but rather patience and love. It's a prayer both for myself and for the patient, for peace of heart.

Milton: There's absolutely no conflict between asking God for healing while also taking action using a tool like medicine. In the Lord's Prayer we ask for our daily bread, but the fact that we've prayed for our food doesn't keep us from planting crops and cooking in order to put meals on the table. We do both: pray and take action.

Plough: *What about sicknesses that involve both a physical component and an emotional or even spiritual component?*

medical care they needed, from routine checkups to the ups and downs of childhood illnesses. For example, when their toddler suddenly had a fever of 105 degrees, Ria called the nurse on duty, who in turn called one of the doctors, who arrived five minutes later at their apartment. When this same child's fever refused to budge and it was ten p.m., a nurse was assigned to care for him through the night until it was clear he was out of

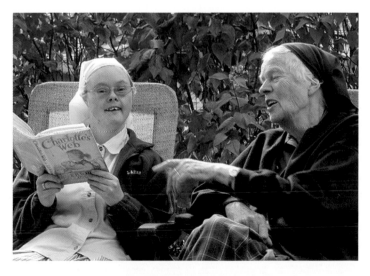

With my daughter Iris

Milton: Well, every illness or health complaint has what you might call a spiritual or emotional or psychiatric aspect – whether it's a headache, asthma, cancer, or a serious infection. A person's attitude toward an illness makes all the difference in the world. We may of course need medical help to get over the problem, but we can't neglect the inner, emotional, spiritual side to it.

> ## "We can't abolish pain. It's part of life, especially as you get older."
>
> *Monika Mommsen*

Monika: Chronic headaches or chronic pain often belong to the category we're talking about – the tests come out normal, we can't identify what's going on, and we may not find a drug. Then we have to find a way to help such patients without labeling or mistrusting them. For them, this may involve learning to accept the pain, which is not an easy thing. We need to stand by them and believe them, because we don't know their pain.

Of course mental disorders are often not exclusively medical in nature. I'm reminded of one patient of mine, a young girl with anorexia, who definitely had medical issues that we treated. Ultimately, though, the most important thing I could do for her was tell her that I believed in her but that she had to be the one to make the decision to overcome her disease – nobody could do it for her. When she finally could do this, she made big steps forward in her health.

One's attitude to life and to one's ailments is extremely important. We can't abolish pain. It's part of life, especially as you get older.

Facing the End of Life

Plough: *You've accompanied dozens of people as they face death. How do you approach telling a person that he or she doesn't have long to live?*

Milton: First and foremost, you need to be open and honest. We never lie to the patient.

Monika: And actually, we try to start that honest conversation earlier, before any diagnosis. When patients come for their routine checkup at age seventy or seventy-five, I will talk to them about the end of life. I'll ask, "Have you ever talked with your spouse or family about your wishes? Have you thought what

---

PATIENT PERSPECTIVE, *continued*

danger. On another occasion their adventurous six-year-old cyclist fell from his new wheels and lacerated the inside of his cheek. They called the dentist (a community member) and met her in the clinic ten minutes later for oral suturing. Money can't buy this type of care – only community can.

Of course, community means giving oneself and surrendering everything for the sake of others, so although I am now very much on the receiving end, I have years of service behind me. In 1957, I gave up a career as the director of a kindergarten – complete with holidays in Rimini and Vienna – to embrace a life of personal poverty and obedience, and the years since have not been without their challenges. But I knew I had found the pearl of great price and gladly gave everything for it. I truly believe this form of community is an expression of the kingdom of God, of how he wants us to care for one another. It is my prayer that more will follow in the footsteps I may soon leave. ⤳

To read the story of Dorli Albertz's daughter Iris, see Erna Albertz's "Pursuing Happiness" in Plough's *Autumn 2016 issue.*

you want us to do if you suddenly become unable to communicate because of a stroke or heart attack? Do you want treatment in hospital, comfort care at home, or some other arrangement? Have you considered a healthcare proxy?" This conversation can lead to a meaningful sharing about life – often they haven't thought about it or wanted to think about it, and this is an opening for them to do so.

Then when someone is diagnosed with a potentially terminal disease like cancer, we'll generally meet with the patient as well as their family and a pastor. In these conversations, as Milton said, honesty is really important – also honesty along the road, especially as you get nearer to the end. Of course, we have no idea when someone will die, and I've become very humble about making a prognosis. But when you can see the end is close, tell the family openly – often they don't realize that they may only have hours or days left.

I experienced it about twelve years ago with an older couple. The husband had almost certainly had a stroke and was very agitated; we couldn't communicate with him anymore. I sat down with the wife and said, "I think your husband is dying." She had such a shock, and then she said, "Thank you, thank you so much. I had no idea. And now I'm really going to spend every minute I can with him." A week later he was gone.

Milton: It's so easy for doctors to get wrapped up in the lab numbers and data, reports and consultations, phone calls and plans, treatments and drug doses; we can get so wrapped up in that, we forget to tell the spouse, "She is dying."

Plough: *What's the place of palliative care?*

Milton: It is different in every case, but we try to consider with the patient prayerfully: What

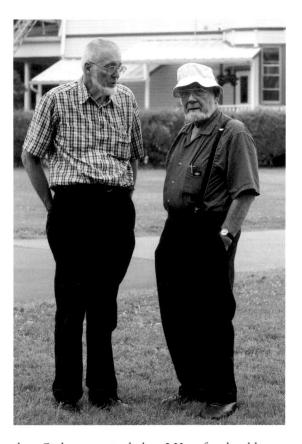

Milton Zimmerman with a long-time friend and patient

does God want us to do here? How far should we go in pursuing aggressive treatments? If there are some good choices, we'll go for them. But at a certain point, one of the jobs of the family doctor is to help the patient discern when a course of treatment could end up being more hurtful than helpful. The patient makes the decision, but it's our job to give them the information they need.

I see some of our poor neighbors getting all kinds of invasive treatments at the hospital that are so fruitless and futile, and I just ache for the unnecessary pain they have to go through in order to die. To what extent does the profit motive on the part of the medical industry play a role here? You wish it wouldn't, you hope it doesn't, but the fact is that many of these desperate treatments are moneymakers.

Monika: It's also not the case that choosing palliative care over treatment amounts to "giving up." On the contrary, recent research suggests that often cancer patients who choose palliative care live longer and better than people who get chemo. Whether a patient decides to pursue treatment such as chemo or surgery or to forego it, I will support them equally.

In the end, as the New Testament tells us, death is the final enemy. All of us will have to face it one day. When the moment comes, it's vitally important to surround the person with peace – peace between us as caregivers and patient, peace in the patient's family, and peace in the community around them. If it's someone who has lived a full life, it can be one of the most wonderful experiences, as difficult as it is.

"You need to learn to look at the whole person, not just the medical issue."

Monika Mommsen

Milton: That is so true. To be present at such a moment enlarges my life, my love, my love for Jesus. I'll never forget a patient who died of lung cancer. On his last morning he looked out the window and saw Venus, the morning star. His son and I pointed it out to him: "Look at the morning star, how bright it is today!" And he looked over and saw it, and smiled, and died. Just like that.

How to Be a Good Doctor

Plough: How have you changed in your approach to practicing medicine?

Milton: I've learned that serving people because you love them includes and surpasses all ideals of professionalism and humanist ethics. Too often, professionalism is a little like diplomacy: diplomacy is knowing how to tell lies politely, and in a similar way professionalism is caring for your patients as though you love them. Well, gosh, if you really do love them, you both fulfill and surpass professional standards.

Monika: I agree. When I started medical school, my father wrote me that I should do it totally as a service, in the same humility shown by the example of Jesus washing his disciples' feet. Being a doctor should have nothing to do with one's own ego.

Listening is really important. I've learned the most about mental illness from my patients – to understand what it's like to suffer from depression. I had a woman in her forties who was bipolar and she told me what it felt like – a much better description than from a textbook.

I take much more time with my patients than I did at first. I try to have more compassion too. Don't be so quick to judge them. Believe in the patient. Believe in what he or she is saying and asking about, even though it may be clear that it's not actually a medical need.

Plough: What advice would you give to medical students preparing to practice medicine today?

Milton: Learn from your patients. Sixty-five years ago I was told in the second year of medical school: "Spend as much time as you can on the ward with patients. Don't just get wrapped up in books." That's still the case, though it has been forgotten in some places.

Second, don't be afraid to practice medicine in the context of faith – that opens up more doors and possibilities for healing than trying to practice medicine without faith. So have faith, pray, study the Bible as well as your textbooks, and don't let technology become a barrier between you and the patient. Work with the family, work with the pastor and the church – the church community can be a fantastic web of social support.

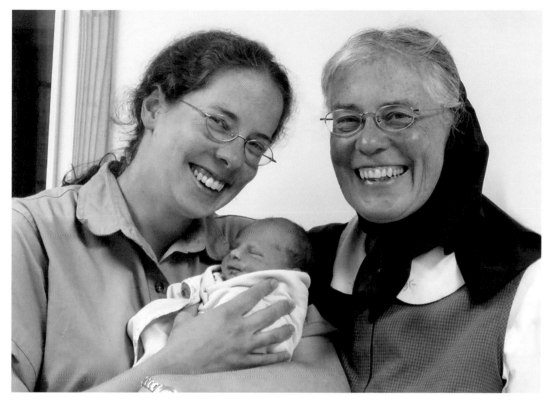

Monika Mommsen with a mother and newborn

Monika: Humility is essential. When you get out of medical school, you're young and full of energy – and you've also had a lot of arrogance pumped into you, especially if you've done well academically. You'll have to shed that pride, because humility brings compassion. You need to learn to look at the whole person, not just the medical issue. There's so much more to a person than the medical side of things: the soul and the spirit, the whole social aspect of family.

And also: have fun. For instance, when someone comes with unexplained chronic pain: first of all, you have to believe the patient – but then, find humor! When they leave your office, they should go encouraged. I had one woman with a long-term mental illness, and my one goal each appointment was to have a laugh together. Another patient, an older woman with advancing Alzheimer's, was my neighbor, so I saw her every day. At times she was very agitated, but if you could

find something to laugh about, it always broke through the barriers of her disease.

Practicing medicine is an enormous privilege: to accompany somebody, to enter into their lives in a way that very few people can, except maybe a pastor. The longer I've done it, the more I've loved it. And I think I'm very lucky to have practiced all these years in a community that supports me in that.

Milton: In caring for someone, we as doctors are only helping along a process of healing that God is doing. Knowing that changes our attitude to our work – it's what gives medicine its value. ⤳

Interview by Peter Mommsen on May 22, 2018.

> ## "We as doctors are only helping along a process of healing that God is doing."
> *Milton Zimmerman*

On Being Ill

VIRGINIA WOOLF

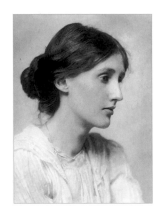

THERE IS, let us confess it (and illness is the great confessional) a childish outspokenness in illness; things are said, truths blurted out, which the cautious respectability of health conceals. About sympathy for example; we can do without it. That illusion of a world so shaped that it echoes every groan, of human beings so tied together by common needs and fears that a twitch at one wrist jerks another, where however strange your experience other people have had it too, where however far you travel in your own mind someone has been there before you – is all an illusion. We do not know our own souls, let alone the souls of others. Human beings do not go hand in hand the whole stretch of the way. There is a virgin forest, tangled, pathless, in each; a snow field where even the print of birds' feet is unknown. Here we go alone, and like it better so. Always to have sympathy, always to be accompanied, always to be understood would be intolerable. But in health the genial pretence must be kept up and the effort renewed – to communicate, to civilize, to share, to cultivate the desert, educate the native, to work by day together and by night to sport. In illness this make-believe ceases. Directly the bed is called for, or, sunk deep among pillows in one chair, we raise our feet even an inch above the ground on another, we cease to be soldiers in the army of the upright; we become deserters. They march to battle. We float with the sticks on the stream; helter skelter with the dead leaves on the lawn, irresponsible and disinterested and able, perhaps for the first time for years, to look round, to look up – to look, for example, at the sky.

Source: "On Being Ill," *The Criterion*, January 1926.

Virginia Woolf (1882–1941) was a British novelist, essayist, and editor.

On Eternal Health

TERESA DE CARTAGENA

Translated by Catherine Addington

Teresa de Cartagena was a fifteenth-century Cistercian nun and writer from Burgos, Spain, who lost her hearing in early adulthood. Her first known work, Grove of the Infirm, *is a spiritual reflection on deafness.*

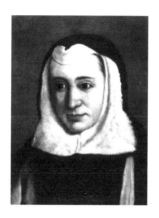

To WHAT supper does my suffering strive to bring me? I believe without a doubt that it is the one of which it is written: "Blessed are those called to the supper of the Lamb." Divine generosity invites all to this blessed feast, but suffering grabs the infirm by their cloak and makes them enter by force. And so it says in the parable that our Lord gives in the Gospel about that man who prepared a great feast and invited many guests, and when it was time to eat, he sent out his servant to inform them that everything was ready. Being occupied with various tasks, or rather with nonsense, they excused themselves from coming; and so the indignant host told his servant, "Go out then to the plazas and markets. Make all the infirm, lame, and weak people that you find come and fill up my house." And he did not say, "Tell them to come," like with the first guests, but rather, "Make them come." And so it seems that the infirm are brought by force to the magnificent feast of eternal health, because their suffering grabs them by the cloak and makes them enter through the door of good works; for if we do not enter through that door, we will not be able to reach the greatest heights of honor, which is to be seated at the table of divine generosity. O blessed convent of the infirm! Of them, I say, who enter willingly where suffering brings them by force, and do not choose to remain in the street.

THEREFORE if suffering afflicts us, let us persevere for the sake of the goodness and honor it promises us; and I know of no greater honor nor dignity in this life than the perfection and virtue that infirmity purifies and refines. . . . Sufferings and afflictions love us, let us love them; health and prosperity reject us, let us reject them for God's sake. . . . It seems to me there are six dishes of which all of us who endure suffering should partake: distressed sadness, enduring

Catherine Addington is a doctoral student of Spanish at the University of Virginia.

patience, bitter contrition, honest and frequent confession, devout prayer, and perseverance in good works. And of these six dishes, and those like them, we may eat without fear; and though they may seem somewhat bitter to our taste, it is necessary that they be so. For few sick people enjoy their diet, but it is beneficial and fortifying nonetheless. So let us desire what is bitter, since what is sweet does not want us; for what human senses perceive as bitter on the palate becomes sweetness for the soul. And I do not know why we infirm should want anything from this world that surrounds us, since we will not find anything in it that wishes us well. Its pleasures detest us, health abandons us, friends forget us, relatives resent us, and even a mother becomes angry with her sick daughter, and a father abhors a son who takes up space in the house with his interminable suffering. And it is no wonder that this should be so, for the sick person comes to abhor and resent himself. Let us not suffer such hunger for worldly things but reach for what is closest at hand, that which is spiritual and healthy for the soul. . . . So let us forsake what forsakes us, and desire only him who desires us, and love only him who gives us these sufferings, so that we might abandon the world and love him who loves us. And that is, without a doubt, the true Father, the loving Father, the only one who never resents our crosses. It is he who heals our infirmities, who keeps us from stumbling and delivers us from danger, who will crown us with great mercies. He will bring our desires to good ends and will renew our youth like an eagle. So let us who are dying of hunger for bodily health in this foreign land search instead for him with fervent desire, for in him we will find true repose, in which our temporal, human sadness will become eternal, spiritual joy. But in the aforementioned things,

patience should reign, for if patience does not rule the convent of the infirm, all our suffering will be fruitless.

THE CAUSE of our sufferings and travails can be attributed to our own sins and the very condition of our human weakness, but on another level it is possible and necessary to observe that if sickness only came because of sinfulness or weakness, neither would the just be subject to it nor would the unjust ever be free of it. But we know this is not so, for though we are all sinful and human, some of us are inflicted with infirmities and plagues while others, in fact the majority, spend their lives free from such adversity. Therefore we cannot doubt that there is a more immediate cause for sickness, and that is the intention or healthy end to which God orders our sufferings, which we cannot deny is good and ultimately for our great benefit, for whoever desires our good loves us. And whoever, in addition to desiring and wanting our good, gives us the ability to realize it – his great love for us shines forth all the more. And what else are infirmities and bodily sufferings, if we consider them carefully or rather tolerate them virtuously, but a sure way to seek and find the most direct path to our salvation? Because there is no straight path to paradise other than the endurance of anguish and tribulation, and by this narrow path we find our wide, spacious, eternal rest. . . . And if the saints could not bypass this path to get to heaven, how do we sinners expect to follow them without enduring trials? ⤜

Source: translated from *Arboleda de los enfermos* (Real Academia Española, 1967).

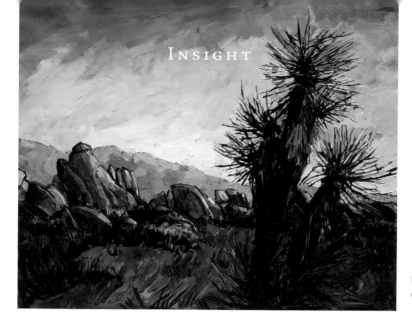

INSIGHT

Erin Hanson,
Cactus Rainbow

Our Task Is to Live

CHRISTOPH FRIEDRICH BLUMHARDT

Sickness is part of the work of death, and death is ultimately a consequence of sin. Destruction of any kind is disorder. It does not belong to life. There is nothing natural about sickness, nothing beneficial; it is something oppressive and contrary to life. Death in the last analysis is a punishment, a punitive power. It is an enemy – indeed, the last enemy!

This is why Jesus calls his church to fight the forces of death. It is no wonder that nursing homes and hospitals originated in the Christian community. We dare not give up on those who are sick and dying, for it belongs to our human dignity and calling to nurture life. Jesus did not say, "Don't bother about what happens to your life." No, he calls himself the resurrection and the life. "The one who believes in me will live, even though they die" (John 11:25).

Therefore, live and resist the spirit of death. Take courage, no matter how much you have to suffer. Protest against death. It is your human task to live! The judgment against our life is now lifted through Christ. Through him everlasting life can flow into us, and we can overcome our fallen existence. This temporal life, cursed by death, need no longer play the tyrant. ➤

From The God Who Heals: Words of Hope for a Time of Sickness *(Plough, 2016).* plough.com/godwhoheals

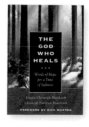

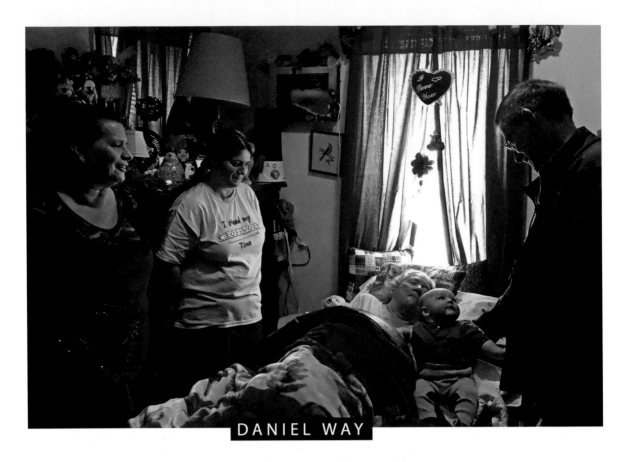

DANIEL WAY

Adirondack Doctor
The Humanity of Rural Medicine

Visiting a patient in her last days

I am an old-school family physician who has spent the last thirty-eight years tending to the population of Hamilton County in the center of upstate New York's Adirondack Park. Hamilton County features the lowest population density of any county in the eastern United States, at 2.6 people per square mile. The people are rugged, stoic, and self-reliant. For economic and geographic reasons, providing health care to them is an ongoing challenge.

Devoting my life's work to practicing rural family medicine in the Adirondacks has been a very rewarding experience. It is true that choosing that path meant placing myself in the lower end of the earnings bracket for my specialty, which is itself one of the least profitable fields in medicine. But my rewards, while less tangible, cannot be bought with money. In the hamlets of North Creek and Indian Lake, I have been able to experience the traditional role of town doctor, where I know almost everyone and almost everyone knows me.

This is especially true when caring for the elderly and infirm who cannot or will not leave their homes. Although they are

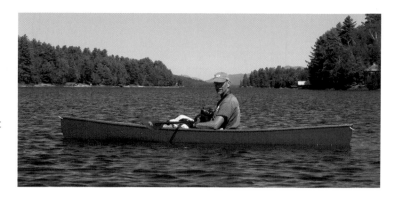

time-consuming, I dedicate one day every two weeks to doing home visits throughout my practice territory, often driving 100 to 150 miles to visit six to ten patients who are too elderly, frail, or ill to travel. I have discovered that this can be a very spiritual experience, especially when the person's medical needs no longer include aggressive or hospital-based care. We can focus on maintaining the individual's comfort, reliving old times, giving reassurance, preserving the patient's dignity, and making sure all concerns are being addressed. I often feel more like a member of the clergy than the medical profession, and it makes me realize how much the two professions have in common.

Having been in practice for three decades, I have witnessed the digitalization, hyper-specialization, over-regulation, and dehumanization of medical care. I have seen fellow physicians retiring from the profession they once loved years earlier than they had planned after succumbing to compassion fatigue, the medical equivalent of battle fatigue known to veterans of armed conflict. It is a sad irony that while the miracles of medical research have enhanced the tools of my trade to an extent I would have thought impossible thirty years ago, the intrusion of the managed care and medical malpractice industries has created such a burden on physicians that, for many of us, the flame of passion for helping our fellow man that was ignited in our youth has burned down prematurely.

In my case, the 9,400-square-mile Adiron-dack Park has become hallowed ground. When I feel stressed, I climb a mountain or get in my carbon-fiber canoe, and head for one of the thousands of ponds, lakes, and streams in the Adirondacks to reconnect with nature. Personal crises seem much less important when I am standing on a mountain summit or floating across a tranquil pond, surrounded by wilderness in every direction. There I can fill my brain (and my camera) with images of the heavenly landscape. The view reminds me how insignificant we are in the grand scheme of things, and why my professional work is so satisfying.

Later in my career it dawned on me that my Adirondack patients were at least as picturesque as the landscape, and that our relationship allowed for very natural, close portraits. And if I could write something about the patients – about their health, our relationships, or their own life stories – the impact of the visual image would be compounded. I was driven by a sense that their lives, hidden away in the folds of the mountains, testified to a dignity and courage that ought to be known beyond their own circle. If they would be willing to share the story written in their faces, I wanted to put it within the pages of a book to live on after they were gone.

As I drive over the mountain lanes, sometimes the camera captures a scene that looks like a Monet painting. Other times it is

The author on Long Lake in his Red Rocket

Daniel Way, MD, has written three books about his work as a primary care physician in the Adiron-dacks. Some stories in this essay are adapted from All in a Day's Work *and* Never a Dull Moment. *Learn more at* danielway.com.

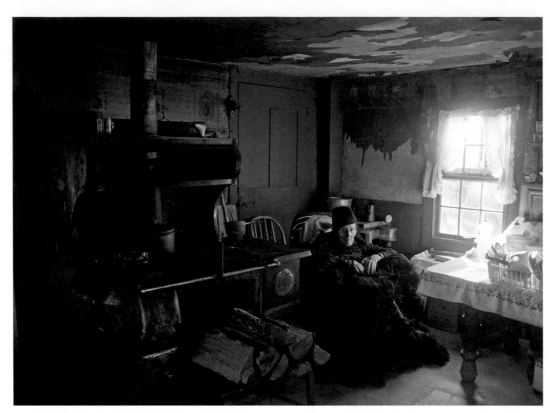

Photography by Daniel Way, unless otherwise noted.

Frank Lillibridge in his Thurman farmhouse

a portrait of a patient that looks like it could have been from the previous century.

Frank Lillibridge was the last master of Maple Grove Farm in Thurman. He grew up in the days when muscles, not machines, performed labor, and men worked on communal projects like cutting hay. His journals vividly portray a life that echoes the farm and forest seasons. In the winter he wrote of hunting and trapping rabbit, raccoon, fox, and muskrat. Each spring, the family tapped four or five hundred sugar maples. Time hardly seemed to touch the farm, or Frank himself, for that matter. An only child, he never married, and stayed true to his land and farm after the deaths of his parents.

Age snuck up on him; he came into my care when he was hospitalized for hypothermia. One cold, rainy day, he went out to dump ashes from the wood stove and fell. He lay outside all night till his neighbor found him the next morning and called the ambulance. Beyond his immediate injuries, he was so stooped, arthritic, and unsteady that I was convinced he would never return to the farm. But when offered a bed in a nursing home, he said simply, "I'll be all right at home, and that's where I'm goin'." His friends took him back to Thurman, where he not only lived for another three years, but regained enough strength to go back to "cuttin' and splittin' a little wood."

The last time I visited him, he asked me if I'd noticed the big maple out in the yard. Of course I had; it was a giant from another era, towering over his house. "I took sap from that tree for over fifty years, and people ask me, 'Why don't you cut it down?' Well, I stopped making syrup when Dad got to be ninety, and I had plenty of other trees for wood. I figured somebody else might want to make syrup from it someday, so I left it for them, whoever they might be."

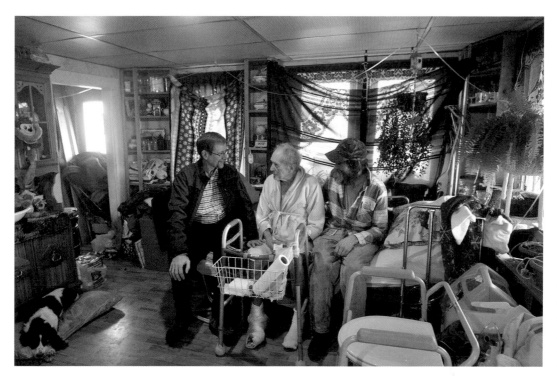

The author visiting Clarence Bateman and his son Joseph

The two-hundred-year-old Bateman farmhouse is located in rural Johnsburg under the shadow of Crane Mountain, whose massive granite slopes shield the adjacent valley from modern life. Clarence "Bud" Bateman has lived here for eighty-odd years, sixty-five of them shared with his wife, Jean. They had nine children, most of whom have families of their own and devote what time they can to helping their parents.

Their youngest son, Joseph, has been the only one who could move in to provide round-the-clock care. A natural jack-of-all-trades, Joe has worked various jobs over the years as a logger, excavator, gravel hauler, and stone mason. But as a young man Joe had problems of his own. When I first met him ten years earlier, he wasn't even taking care of himself. The casual observer might have dismissed him as just another bachelor mountain man in the habit of spending what little he had on alcohol. That would have been an accurate assessment – then. But he had the guts to ask

for help. "I wanted to quit drinking because it was a choice of whether I wanted to live or die," he says now in his matter-of-fact manner. He needed a safe haven to clean up his life, and his folks needed someone with dedication, determination, and a gift for improvisation. Fortunately, Joe has these traits in abundance. Once committed, Joe quickly learned the skills of a caregiver. He has been responsible for his parents' total care for years now.

Caring for a loved one is among the most selfless acts that can be imagined. I have seen

Joseph Bateman

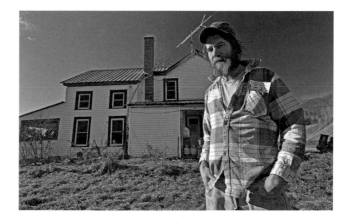

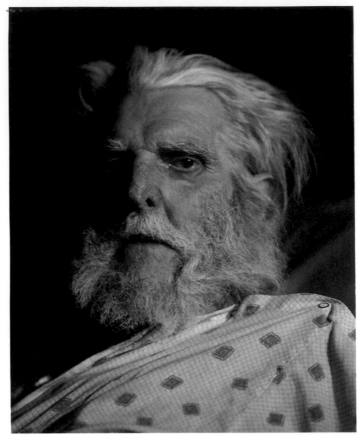

Jesse
Warren

many examples of caregivers who suffered serious physical, emotional, social, and financial hardships. Joe is acutely aware of this. Yet he continues to tend to his parents' needs, with no predictable endpoint. "I know Dad doesn't want to go back to the hospital or live out his days in a nursing home," he told me, "so I'll take care of him as long as I have to. I have no regrets – I'd do it all again – but there's times I want to take a long walk, or step back, and count to ten, or ten thousand. . . . I still go four-wheeling and hunting just to get away for a while. When I get back home, I know I have to keep the firewood up, the house warm, the laundry moving. . . . I don't know how long I'm gonna be able to keep this place going, but we'll think of something."

Anyone who understands the personal sacrifices Joe is making can appreciate the determination he must have to keep going. And he hasn't touched a drop of alcohol in many years. He has my highest respect.

I only came to know Jesse Warren very briefly when he was hospitalized for treatment of advanced pulmonary emphysema. Struck by his piercing eyes and flowing white mane, I had the sensation that I was in the presence of the abolitionist John Brown. Jesse was in very frail health, requiring oxygen whenever he moved around. He had spent most of the last few months in the hospital, and his prognosis for recovery was poor. Yet he was interested in my interest in him, and wistfully spoke to me about his long life as a farmer in Washington County. I asked him if he would mind my taking his photo, and he graciously agreed. It took several days to get prints made for him. When I mailed them to his home address, they were returned as undeliverable. When I went back to that hospital to see if he was still there, I learned that Jesse had died.

When the emergency physician called me out of a sound sleep at two a.m. for a patient experiencing severe diabetic ketoacidosis, I had no idea who I was about to meet. After four hours, six liters of IV fluid, over eighty units of insulin, and a lot of work from a dedicated team, Winifred Young began to come out of her coma. As she tried to orient herself, her eyes locked on mine, and she whispered, "Are you my doctor?"

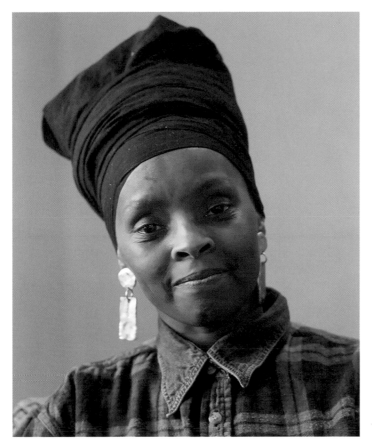

Did you know that you are beautiful?"

I glanced over my shoulder to see whom she was addressing, but no one else was there to take the credit. Winnie's family has been in this area for generations. Her ancestors were among the first five black families to settle in the city of Albany in the 1880s. I have never seen her again. But I will never forget the grace she taught me.

Winifred Young

Albert and Eleanor Alger lived along the Hudson River below The Glen, in a one-room cabin lit by a single sixty-watt bulb and heated by an ancient wood stove. In earlier years, Eleanor had made a career as a circus performer, while Albert was once a lumberjack. They took care of each other in their tiny home through years of debilitating illness. When I asked Eleanor how they survived with almost no visible means of support, she replied lightheartedly, "We're not poor, we just don't have any money!" That their life was simple and by modern standards, very difficult, was obvious to me. But to them, they were at home, together, in a place of welcome. They didn't ask for more.

I would never call this work easy. But in return for my efforts, I have the knowledge that I've been able to make a difference in the lives of my neighbors. I have become an integral part of the community, and all the respect, affection, and appreciation I have shown my patients has been showered back upon me many times over. ➷

"Yes," I answered.

"What's your name?"

"My name is Daniel Way. It's good to see you feeling better." With all the strength she had, she whispered, "I *am* feeling better. God bless you, Daniel Way." Then she fell asleep.

Her words uplifted me, as if a window had been opened, letting in a draft of fresh air. A moment before, I had been exhausted and in need of a large infusion of caffeine, but now I felt inexplicably energized.

More conversations with Winnie left me in awe. When I learned that she had been diabetic for over half her life, yet had never suffered any of the significant organ damage so common to the disease, I asked her if she thought her joyous attitude to life might have helped her physical health. "My Momma gave that to me when I was very young. She always told me to love myself and see the beauty in other people.

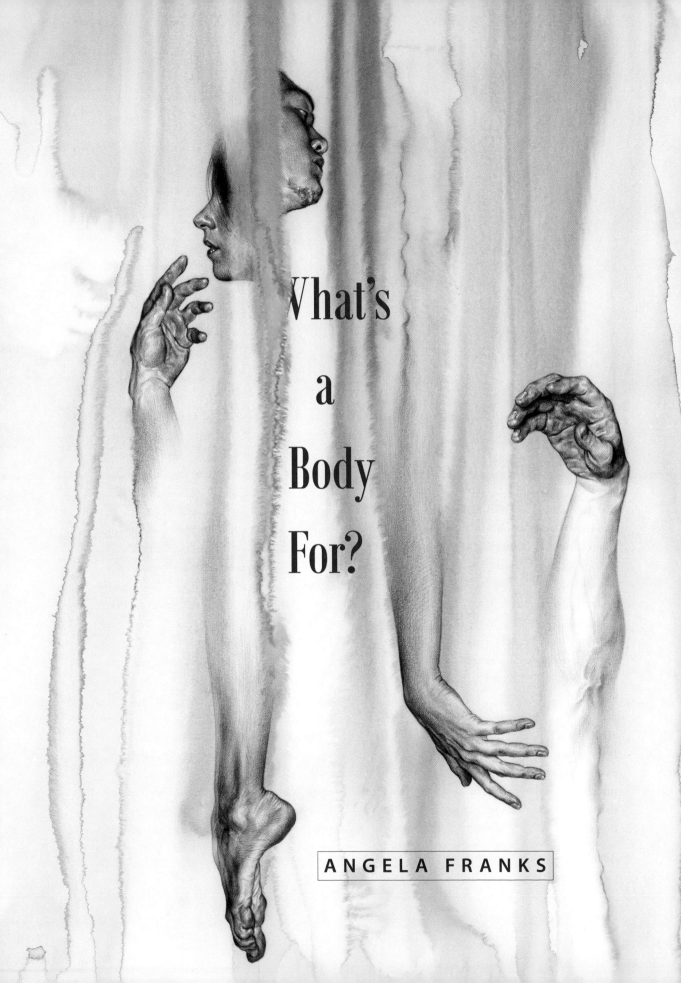

What's a Body For?

ANGELA FRANKS

Item 1: a cover story in *Christianity Today* about evangelical Christians who rent out their wombs as reproductive surrogates, in order to help those who cannot conceive;

Item 2: an essay in *First Things* by an evangelical professor lamenting the heterodoxy of her Christian students, who cheerfully call their bodies "meat suits" while doubting the resurrection of the flesh;

Item 3: an article in *The Wall Street Journal* by a biologist decrying the evolutionary "botch" that is the human body.

Each of these items crossed my field of vision in the space of a few weeks this spring. And I'm not even counting the continuing drip of #MeToo fallout. Clearly, the body is a vexed site of controversy.

What is the body for, anyway? The materialist has one answer: for nothing in particular. It's just an accidental confluence of DNA, fluky environmental factors, and the inexorable march of time, in which change is the only constant. Don't get too attached to this iteration of humanity, because it won't last.

Many of today's Christians have another answer: it's for getting me to heaven. The evangelical surrogates use their bodies as a useful tool of ministry to infertile couples. The students negotiate the body's demands through spiritual damage-control. In both cases, the body is a potential minefield of desire and use-values.

But mastered by whom? Who is the "I" that is going to heaven? The disbelief in the resurrection of the flesh reveals that many Christians do not think that their "I" includes their bodies. The "I" is the soul, some kind of ghostly substance that stands over and above the body. And yet, as Pope Benedict XVI says in *Deus Caritas Est,* "It is neither the spirit alone nor the body alone that loves: it is man, the person, a unified creature composed of body and soul, who loves."

The Gnosticism of many contemporary Christians is only the latest iteration of the heresy that has parasitically attached itself to Christianity from the very beginning. Gnosticism has many permutations, but one common thread is the conviction that the material world

Watercolor and colored pencil artwork by Wanjin Gim

Angela Franks, PhD, is a theologian, speaker, writer, and mother of six. She is a professor of theology at Saint John's Seminary in Boston.

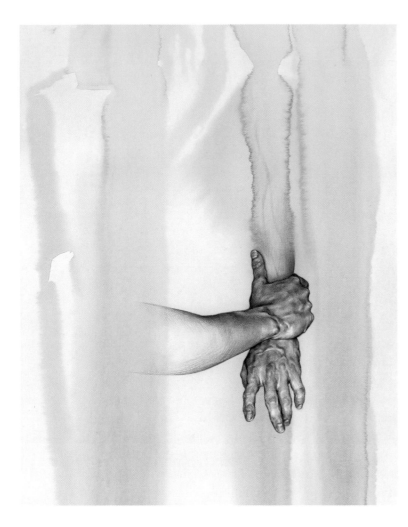

Artwork by
Wanjin Gim

(John 21), and the insistence that the beloved disciple has seen and touched Jesus (1 John 1).

The delicate approach John takes with the word "flesh" (*sarx*) indicates the balancing act Christianity had to achieve vis-à-vis the body. On the one hand, as 1 John 2:16 emphasizes, "For all that is in the world, the lust of the flesh and the lust of the eyes and the pride of life, is not of the Father but is of the world." The flesh has its lusts, and these are "of the world." Both "flesh" and "world" can be morally neutral terms in the New Testament, referring simply to the body and to the whole of creation respectively. But they can also, as here, refer to the desires of the human being when cut off from God. These desires lead man to try to make his home in the "world" – that is, without God.

has its source in some evil power. Contrary to the Gnostics of the second century AD, who "represent all material substance to be formed from three passions, namely, fear, grief, and perplexity," and "deny that He [Christ] assumed anything material, since indeed [they believed that] matter is incapable of salvation," Irenaeus argued that the material world has its source in one good God.

The Gnostic ideas that Irenaeus battled were challenged already in the Johannine writings, which emphasized – to the point of uncouthness – the raw physicality of Jesus' body and commands: the eating of his body (John 6), the holes in his hands and side (John 20), the breakfast he solicitously cooks

On the other hand, the Johannine literature also emphasizes that Jesus is the Word made flesh (John 1:14). The denial of the Incarnation ("Jesus Christ has come in the flesh") is equated to the spirit of the Antichrist (1 John 4). Flesh is not an evil principle but rather, incomplete. It requires God and his grace to become what it should be. As with the flesh, so too with the world: "For the creation waits with eager longing for the revealing of the sons of God . . . because the creation itself will be set free from its bondage to decay and obtain the glorious liberty of the children of God" (Rom 8:19, 21).

As Irenaeus said against the Gnostics of the

second century, salvation centers around the flesh: God created the flesh of man, which the Son assumes in the Incarnation, all so that he might save the flesh of man. Tertullian states this idea straightforwardly: *caro salutis cardo,* the flesh is the hinge of salvation.

First Corinthians 6:19–20 develops this anthropology by giving it a pneumatological angle: "Do you not know that *your body* is a temple of the Holy Spirit within you, which you have from God? You are not your own; you were bought with a price. So glorify God in your body." This language restates the earlier exhortation at 1 Corinthians 3:16–17: "Do you not know that *you* are God's temple and that God's Spirit dwells in you? . . . For God's temple is holy, and that temple you are." Note how easily Paul moves between "your body" and "you."

But more can be said on this point. The holy things of God are owed reverence, and this includes the body-temple (1 Thess. 4:4; 1 Cor. 12:22–25). The proper attitude toward the body, as a temple of the Spirit, is that of "piety," traditionally one of the seven gifts of the Holy Spirit taken from Isaiah 11:1–3 ("the Spirit of the fear of the Lord"). We don't owe our body mere toleration; we owe it reverence.

All well and good. But still the question remains: Why do we have bodies in the first place? The compelling simplicity of contemporary Gnosticism provides one answer: because a rival and evil god is in control of the material world. As one Vatican document recently summarized Pope Francis's warnings, neo-Gnosticism "presumes to liberate the human person from the body and from the material universe, in which traces of the provident hand of the Creator are no longer found, but only a reality deprived of meaning, foreign to the fundamental identity of the person, and easily manipulated by the interests of man." Against such contemporary Gnosticism, John Paul II provided another answer: the body expresses the person.

This answer was spelled out in a series of remarkable talks from 1979–1984 and popularized as the "theology of the body." In it, John Paul II argues that we have bodies in order to make visible what is invisible: namely, our persons. My "I" is not separable from my body, but neither is it reducible to it. My body is the exterior expression of that interior personal reality that Scripture names the "heart," the most common anthropological term in the Old Testament, according to one scholar. When Jesus says that "everyone who looks at a woman lustfully has already committed adultery with her in his heart" (Matt. 5:28), he is reminding us that the body's look reveals the person. As John Paul II puts it, the "look" is the "threshold of the person."

This proposal is dramatically countercultural. Take, for example, transgenderism, which requires that there be no intrinsic link between the body and the person. For the trans person, the body first needs to be modified technologically in order to be capable of personal expressiveness. This process often coopts the medical profession, which exists to heal sick bodies. Transgenderism instead demands that it surgically manipulate healthy bodies, often by the removal of healthy organs. Likewise, the reproductive surrogate views her womb as a detachable tool, such that she need not *be* the mother of whatever child happens to be residing in it temporarily.

The body's job of expressing the person is nonsense to a materialist, who refuses the

> # We don't owe our bodies mere toleration; we owe them reverence.

Artwork used by permission of the artist

very idea of an interior to man. It's matter all the way down. The earnest Christian Gnostic believes there is an interior, but it is the real "I," and hence the body is somehow detachable from it. Both positions cannot integrate body and soul; at best, the two move on parallel tracks, never to meet, like train tracks stretching into infinity. But John Paul II insists that God designed us as an integrated whole, precisely so that we – the only embodied spirits – could make visible his love to the world through our loving.

A corollary of this truth is that the body is never the problem, in the deepest sense of the word. Transgenderism implies that the body's "wrongness" is the problem. For John Paul II, the buck doesn't stop with the body, because the body simply expresses what is in the heart. If the ultimate problem is the body, the solution is technological manipulation of it. If the ultimate problem is the heart, then the solution is conversion. Hence, as John Paul II writes in the theology of the body, the pretense that the body is simply matter to be dominated "threatens the human person for whom the method of 'self-mastery' is and remains specific."

God delights in using matter to express his invisible mystery.

How might this look in real life? Technology can be of service to the body, of course, when it enhances its ability to express a person's self-gift. For example, the birth of my fourth child required an emergency caesarean section, because of placenta previa. Without the C-section, I could have bled to death. Because of that surgical intervention, I was able to continue as a mother to my children. Similarly, my father has a pacemaker, which he needs to keep his heart rhythms regular. Because of that device, he can continue to be a loving husband, father, and grandfather.

The kind of technological manipulation that John Paul II decries is the kind that treats the body as distinct from the person. If the body is simply clay in our hands, why not make it differently gendered? Or make our children as smart and blond as possible through genetic engineering? Or upload our minds to computer databases and discard the body altogether? All of these approaches make the body a problem to be fixed or eliminated.

Why do we make the body into the problem? In part, because of our resentment against its intransigence. Our bodies, when they resist us by getting sick, old, and tired, constantly remind us that the world is not plastic matter responsive to the whims of our freedom. We yearn for a freedom that is not tied to embodiment. "A freedom which claims to be absolute ends up treating the human body as a raw datum, devoid of any meaning and moral values until freedom has shaped it in accordance with its design," John Paul II writes in his encyclical *Veritatis Splendor*. We want to be "light," untrammeled by any limitations outside of our own will.

This worldview harms everyone, but it particularly denigrates women, who have traditionally been connected with what is bodily. It's no accident that myths proposed "Mother Earth," in contrast to the male gods, who were often gods of the air and lightning. Women have always been connected to the earth, to the physical, because of the earth's fruitfulness. As the earth brings forth fruit, likewise women bear the fruit of children.

This primitive view had to be supplemented with a deeper anthropology in Judeo-Christianity, but the basic insight was not denied. A woman's body intrudes into her thoughts;

she cannot ignore it as easily as a man can ignore his. Simone de Beauvoir lamented this intrinsic materiality, the fact that a woman's body is inevitably impacted through childbearing. She envied the airy lightness of the man, "a being who is not given, who makes himself what he is."

As a result, when a culture turns against embodiment, women feel the bite first. Theologian Margaret Harper McCarthy summarizes: "It is the woman's body that opposes her existence as a person. It is therefore ultimately her own body that the woman must resist." The modern age has furthered the interior fracture women sense between themselves and their bodies.

Against this fracture, we can insist that the body's materiality serves a purpose: the body expresses the person. The weight of the body expresses a truth that we might like to forget: namely, that we are made for love and fruitfulness. Because we are made in the image of God, this truth about ourselves is a pale echo of who God is: "He first loved us" (1 John 4:19). Women's bodies, tied as obviously as they are to fruitfulness, have a special role in testifying to the fruitful creativity that is intrinsic to the human person.

The embodied person can testify to this truth in a profound way. In fact, God delights in using matter to express his invisible mystery. "The world is charged with the grandeur of God," writes poet Gerard Manley Hopkins, and in water, bread, wine, oil, and the bodies and words of persons, God expresses and communicates that grandeur in particularly efficacious ways. The visibility of the body is a kind of "primordial sacrament," according to John Paul II, the very foundation of the sacramental order. (Angels don't have sacraments.)

Through the faith and hope bestowed by the sacraments, "we ourselves, who have the first fruits of the Spirit, groan inwardly as we wait for adoption as sons, the redemption of our bodies. For in this hope we were saved" (Rom. 8:23–24). The redemption wrought by Christ penetrates all the way down, even into our bodies. This is an intrinsic part of the Good News we have been commissioned to share. Ultimately, our bodies are for the new heaven and the new earth – that is, for Christ and his kingdom.

As the Second Vatican Council taught, "When we have spread on earth the fruits of our nature and our enterprise . . . according to the command of the Lord and in his Spirit, we will find them once again, cleansed this time from the stain of sin, illuminated and transfigured, when Christ presents to his Father an eternal and universal kingdom." Right now we love and labor by means of our bodies, but these things have eternal weight.

Thus, our bodies are not meat-suits to be discarded or clusters of atoms that will disintegrate and disappear. They are made to last, because God's kingdom will last, taking up from this world all that is good and preserving it. All that is made in and through Christ – including the body – will find its ultimate meaning in him. "My soul longs, yea, faints for the courts of the Lord; my heart and flesh sing for joy to the living God" (Ps. 84:2). ⤳

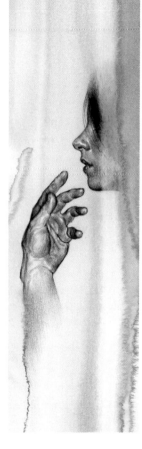

Artwork detail by Wanjin Gim

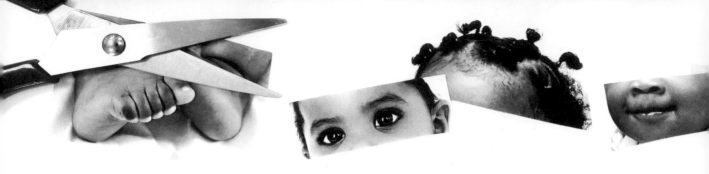

Begotten Not Made

A molecular biologist and priest on CRISPR and designer babies

NICANOR AUSTRIACO

THE HUMAN GENOME consists of twenty-three pairs of chromosomes. These forty-six chromosomes in turn are made up of six billion chemical DNA units called DNA base pairs. Thus, one can visualize a human genome as an encyclopedia of forty-six volumes written with six billion letters.

Thanks to the discovery of CRISPR (Clustered Regularly Interspaced Short Palindromic Repeats), we will conceivably be able to open this genetic encyclopedia to any page and edit any single letter. Shortly after CRISPR's discovery, a cover story in the *Economist* imagined a society where children are designed so that they are born with perfect pitch, 20/20 vision, no baldness, and decreased risk of Alzheimer's, breast cancer, and stroke, to name just a few editable features.

What are we to think about the possibility of genetically engineering future generations? As a Catholic priest who is also an MIT-trained molecular biologist and a moral theologian, I have been privy to many conversations among professional ethicists, biologists, and others that have convinced me that the ethical landscape for CRISPR-based technologies can be summarized best by considering three distinctions.

First, there is the distinction between therapeutic and non-therapeutic gene editing. Therapeutic interventions delay, prevent, or treat disease and disability. Non-therapeutic interventions, on the other hand, seek to promote some good of the individual other than his or her health and well-being, often seeking to enhance the person's access to opportunity, privilege, and power. Think here of proposals to design children who are taller, smarter, or more attractive, specifically because it will give them an advantage in life over their non-designed peers.

Secondly, there is the distinction between somatic cell and germline cell gene editing. The former refers to gene editing of any cells in our body other than our egg or sperm cells, while the latter refers to gene editing of these reproductive cells. Significantly, any changes made to the genomes of somatic cells would not be heritable, while changes made to eggs

Nicanor Austriaco, OP, is a molecular biologist, priest, and professor of biology and theology at Providence College.

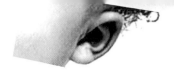

and to sperm would be handed down to future generations.

An example of somatic cell gene editing: Sickle cell disease is caused by a single genetic mutation in the patient's genome, actually a single alphabet change from an "A" to a "T," which causes red blood cells to form an abnormal, sickle shape. These sickle cells can clog a patient's blood vessels, depriving her cells of oxygen, which damages organs, causes severe pain, and often leads to premature death. By correcting the mutation in the blood stem cells back to an "A" and reintroducing these corrected blood stem cells into the patient's bone marrow, physicians could replace her diseased sickle cells with normal round blood cells, curing her of this debilitating ailment. Notably, however, the patient could still bear children who would suffer from sickle cell disease if they inherit her mutated disease gene, precisely because the genome of her germ cells was not edited.

And finally, there is the concept of dignity. I am often asked what it's like to debate bioethics in a pluralistic, post-Christian society. I respond by proposing that most disagreements between faith-based bioethicists and their secular counterparts stem from a fundamental disagreement about the nature of human dignity.

Secular ethicists tend to believe that human dignity is only extrinsic, and can therefore be diminished or lost through pain, suffering, or disability. If human dignity can be lost, it follows that we should be able to modify ourselves in ways that we believe would either advance or preserve our dignity. This conception of dignity is the ethical justification given by those who believe that we should be free to design our children so that our species becomes stronger, smarter, more healthy, more attractive, and therefore more dignified.

In contrast, faith-based ethicists believe that human beings have dignity that can never be diminished or lost. The Judeo-Christian tradition holds that humans have intrinsic dignity, based on the belief that we are made in the image and likeness of God. This dignity thus cannot be lost, from conception until death, no matter the apparent indignities a person suffers.

It is on this that I base my opposition to non-therapeutic gene editing. Children should be welcomed and not designed.

Recently, for my students here at Providence College, I summarized the technological advances, especially CRISPR, that make designer babies possible. Then I asked: "Would it change things if you discovered that you had been designed by your parents?" One student said that she would always wonder if her parents would still have loved her if she had been the way that she was supposed to have been. Another student added that he would forever worry about falling short of the expectations that his parents had when they designed him, and admitted that he would have resented his parents for this. A third student worried that he would hate his parents for making him something that he did not want to be.

My many conversations have convinced me that the debate over designer babies is not really a debate over the use of CRISPR technology. Rather, it is a debate over how we should understand ourselves and our relationships with others. Designing a child makes his sense of self subject to the whims and fancies of another, and undermines his conviction that he is irreplaceably and individually unique, a gift to be cherished and loved by others. For these reasons – and there are many more – children should be begotten and not made.

The End Of Medicine

Euthanasia and the campaign to "take death back"

REUBEN ZIMMERMAN

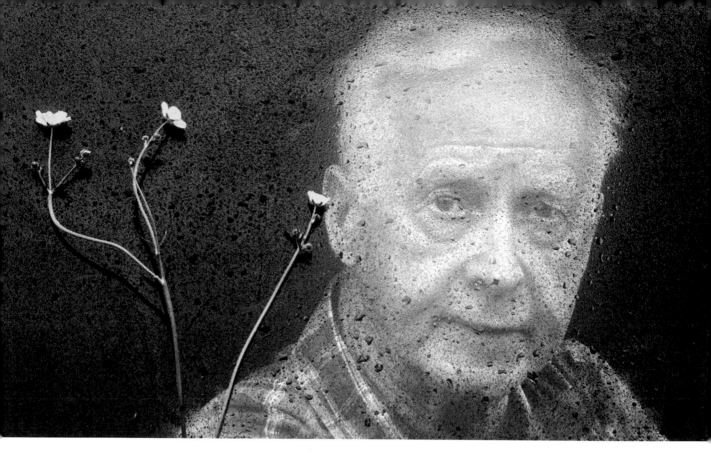

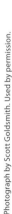

O n May 25, 2017, the *New York Times* published a front page article about a man in British Columbia who planned his own wake – a living wake, that is – and who, after most of his friends had left, succumbed to a lethal injection administered by his doctor.

The article is well-written, and convincing. There is a sick man who doesn't have much longer to live, or who (more accurately) is tired of living with his illness. There are eagle feathers and prayer shawls, and good food and hugs and tears. People light candles and present blessings and talk about "taking death back." But someone is going to be killed, and even the doctor who administers the deadly drugs to the man acknowledges as much. Though "that's not how I think of it," she says adamantly. "It's my job. I do it well."

Other examples abound. There is the story of the elderly couple in Oregon who recently chose to go together: after sixty-six years of marriage, including years as medical missionaries in India, they decided that old age and infirmity – between them, Parkinsonism, heart disease, and cancer – were too much to bear. After their family documented their exit on video, they were duly hailed as brave exemplars of the new way to die.

Untitled,
Scott
Goldsmith

Reuben Zimmerman is a physician assistant who lives and works at Woodcrest, a Bruderhof in Rifton, New York.

Then there is Brittany Maynard, the twenty-nine-year-old woman in California with an inoperable brain tumor whose struggle for the "right" to die led to assisted-suicide legislation there and in other states. Promoted as a hero by the likes of *People* magazine and CNN, she moved to Oregon to obtain the drug cocktail by which she ended her young life.

But it's not just cancer and neuromuscular disability that is driving people to opt out of living. Increasingly, it's depression – "exhaustion" with life – and now, in parts of Europe, even just old age. What is going on, and why?

Who Is Pushing for Euthanasia?

Having cared for the sick and dying for over twenty-five years, I can well understand what drives people to take matters into their own hands. Despite everything modern medicine has to offer, it has not yet conquered death, nor the suffering that sometimes precedes it by decades, and it is not likely that it ever will. Even as we have learned to successfully treat childhood leukemia and eliminate polio and diphtheria, we have not yet found cures for the scourges – arthritis, heart failure, incontinence, or insomnia – that seem to mar old age for so many people, even those who live in the most attractive neighborhoods and who don't have to worry about their finances.

Data from the states where assisted suicide is now legal suggest that people aren't signing up for lethal prescriptions just because they're in pain. Instead, it's because they are afraid of "losing control" – because they are lonely, afraid, or worried that they have become a burden on their caregivers – or simply because they want to do things "their own way." In California, for example, the vast majority of people who have taken their own lives under the new right-to-die law have been well-educated white seniors who were already receiving palliative or hospice care. Almost all of them also had medical insurance, so cost was not necessarily an issue. And in Canada, one doctor who is also a longtime supporter of assisted suicide says that the patients who request his services come from a particular personality type: they tend to be the "doctors, lawyers, captains of industry, and successful business people" who "always get what they want."

Given the spiritual emptiness and materialism that often characterize modern life, along with the presumption that human happiness depends primarily on mobility, independence, and self-determination, it is understandable that we should have come to this place. But if it is understandable, it is also an indictment on those of us who call ourselves Christians. Too often, we have embraced our culture's false gospel that happiness really depends on the absence of inconvenience and suffering. From there, it's a small step to seek to bypass the infirmities of old age and disease by engineering one's own death.

The Place of Bravery

For centuries, human beings fought against death with everything they had. Death was unavoidable, but it was still something to be feared and delayed. Now, however, we are suddenly facilitating it, even embracing it, as a solution to the pain and the problems of living. The reason for the shift, we are told, is that advances in modern medicine, especially life-support technologies that can postpone death indefinitely, have fundamentally changed the moral calculus. The old Hippocratic ban on causing a patient's death must supposedly yield to today's realities.

But even if suicide or euthanasia is described in comforting euphemisms and carried out on a comfortable bed in the privacy of our homes, is it really the solution to these

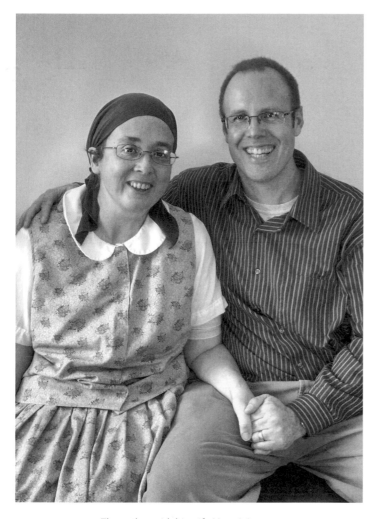

The author with his wife Margrit in 2015

lives were not lived solely for ourselves, but were in some way poured out for others.

It also depends on faith, which the apostle Paul defined as the assurance of things hoped for, and the conviction of things not yet seen. Many people today mock faith as the property of unenlightened zealots. And yet the real enlightenment is to know that with faith, we can boldly enter the realm which in this life we do not see or know. Faith can bring us a peace that surpasses all human understanding, a confidence that the throes of death are overcome not by a syringe of midazolam but by embracing what has been laid on us, trusting that it will not be more than we can endure.

My own wife, Margrit, was an example of such faith. Stricken by small bowel cancer at the age of forty-three, she fought back for twenty-two months until it was clear that she could not win. At that point, she faced death squarely, and with a calm bravery that came from far beyond herself.

Letting go wasn't easy: she was in the prime of life, as were our five children, all between the ages of twelve and nineteen. So she shed tears over missed graduations and weddings, over the grandchildren she would never see, and over the fact that she would leave me a widower at forty-seven. But she also looked back with joy and gratitude at the life she had lived as a wife and mother and nurse: at the many births she had attended, the hundreds of

dilemmas? Those of us who see the body as more than a mass of quivering cells must protest that it is not. If we are spiritual beings, made in the image of God, then our reasons to keep living can never depend completely on physical ability or the absence of discomfort.

All of us long for personal fulfillment, for happiness, and for good health, and we also want our lives to be meaningful. And yet such meaning cannot be measured by the absence of hearing aids and wheelchairs and oxygen tanks; rather, it must result from the knowledge that we have spent our best years in the service of God and our fellow human beings – that our patients she had cared for, and the thousands of lives she had touched, knowingly and unknowingly, over many years.

She was ready to go because she had served, and her years of service to others now allowed her to rest with a sense of peaceful (if humble) accomplishment. Thus when I asked her, weeks before the end, if she was afraid, she could answer, "No, I don't think so. I believe Jesus is coming to fetch me."

We celebrated our twenty-fifth wedding anniversary in December 2014, and by January 2015, she could manage only yogurt and broth. By February it was weak tea, fortified with honey and cream. By March, she was gone. Despite receiving the best care medicine could offer, she still suffered terribly in her last ten days: malignant small bowel obstruction, which invariably leads to vomiting, is one of the most difficult situations palliative medicine experts have to deal with. Still, she never once flinched or complained, and instead radiated peace and love, often through shining eyes, until her last agonizing breath.

She went Home surrounded by her family: her parents, my parents, her siblings, and our children. There was singing, and there were prayers, and plenty of tears, and we prayed often that she might somehow be released, but we never once contemplated pushing things along or taking things into our own hands. Like those willing to await the birth of a baby, we waited for God's moment, knowing that just as those gathered around a laboring woman rejoice when the child bursts out of the womb, those waiting for Margrit in the

world beyond would break into singing when she crossed her Jordan.

She was blessed with a strong faith, and yet it wasn't just her faith that held her through: it was the love of the community to which we belong that carried her, and our family, through the most difficult hours. She received expert medical care, but more than that, she received pastoral care in the form of house calls and prayers, songs and services. From the moment she was diagnosed with cancer, people rallied around her. Children brought flowers, old friends dropped by to reminisce, acquaintances we hardly knew dropped in with baskets of food. But what of the thousands of people who lack such love? And could it be the absence of this love that is driving so many of them to take matters into their own hands?

> It wasn't just her faith that held her through: it was the love of the community to which we belong.

Dying in the Church

In 1651, George Fox, founder of the Quakers, famously told Oliver Cromwell's representatives that he wished to live such a life that would "take away the occasion for war." Might we now dare to live such a life that would take away the occasion for suicide and euthanasia? And if so, what might such a life look like? In an age that prizes autonomy and individualism above everything else, derides accountability, and worships self-sufficiency, creating such a life will be no easy task. But if Christ calls us to bear one another's burdens, can we do anything less?

The hospitals of medieval Europe, in fact, were established as religious communities in which monks and nuns cared for the sick and the dying; the French called them *hôtels-Dieu*, or "hostels of God." By the ninth century,

Charlemagne had ordered cathedrals and monasteries to build their own hospital facilities, some of which survive to this day; the tradition has been carried on by the Catholic Church. Sadly, as medicine evolved into a largely scientific discipline, its original spiritual core, though no less needed today, has largely withered away. Thus people now die attached to machines and monitors that blink and beep, while family and friends, sequestered in plush conference rooms, wait to be called in "when it is all over." Such is the irony of modern medicine: though aiming nobly to eliminate suffering, we have unwittingly abandoned the dying.

If we really want to take death back, we need to bring the dying back into our churches and into our homes. We need to push away those intrusions of medicine that pointlessly serve only to prolong the process of dying, even as we embrace those interventions that do relieve pain and breathlessness and nausea. We need to bring back priests and pastors and music, but most of all, we need to invite God back into the picture and put our trust in him, instead of in those new midwives of death, who, syringes in hand, promise a swift and painless dispatch into the unknown (and unaccompanied) night.

Margrit's dying was not quick or easy, but as I look back on it now, I am certain that it was exactly as God intended it to be. She suffered, and yet bringing God back into the picture does not mean eliminating suffering; it means discovering and learning the only real way to bear it. Thus there was deep spiritual worth in our waiting for God's moment; profound lessons learned from the mystery of not knowing, and of not being in control. We

If we really want to take death back, we need to bring the dying back into our churches and into our homes.

were helpless, and yet at the same time we were cushioned by unseen wings, and even as we grieved we could rejoice as hard hearts were softened, dull consciences stirred, and closed eyes opened.

The ancients believed we could learn something from the dying: that they were stretched between heaven and earth. To the extent that we ourselves resist the urge to meddle with divine timing, there is much we can learn from them still today. In the community where I live and work, almost no one dies in the hospital, much less the ICU. Most, like Margrit, die at home, in their own beds, surrounded by flowers and music and children and singing. They are very ordinary people, and they fear death and disability like anyone else, but the active love that surrounds them helps answer their fears, and the prayers of those who watch with them through long days and even longer nights uphold and strengthen them more powerfully than any carefully titrated medicine. They also do not die alone, and never need to organize their own wakes.

We cannot condemn those who, whether from fear of the future or due to the misery of their condition, decide to end their own lives, but we can point to another way. This is the way of hope in life beyond death and the way of meaning in and through suffering.

The apostle Matthew shows us this way when he describes the suffering of Christ: his very human reaction to it (he prayed for deliverance) and his ultimate obedience and bravery. Incredibly, when hanging on the cross, he refused vinegar mixed with gall, a mixture which historians tell us was supposed to numb the mind and thereby dull pain. He did this so that he could face death with a clear mind: proof that he was laying down his life for us, accepting suffering voluntarily.

In this way is his death an example to those of us who claim to follow him, and in this way will all of us, facing the inevitable pain and infirmity that is our lot, one day be faced with the same choice: to reject and avoid suffering, or to submit to it in God's name – and with his grace allow ourselves to be purified and redeemed through it.

Already in the first century, the apostle Peter exhorted his readers to submit to the discipline of suffering, suggesting that it could serve a holy purpose: "Since therefore Christ suffered in the flesh, arm yourselves also with the same intention, for whoever has suffered in the flesh has finished with sin" (1 Pet. 4:1). Peter goes on to say, "But rejoice insofar as you are sharing Christ's sufferings, so that you may also be glad and shout for joy when his glory is revealed" (1 Pet. 4:13). Paul similarly suggests that we should "boast in our sufferings, knowing that suffering produces endurance" (Rom. 5:3).

The writers of these New Testament passages may have been talking primarily about religious persecution, but, in the end, the subjugation of the body – and the spiritual purification with which we can be blessed as a result – need not depend on the source of our pain. An example of this is Alison Davis, who, as Robert Carle writes, survived a suicide attempt and whose newfound will to live exemplifies the possibility of finding a fruitful and fulfilled life, even when that life has been physically wrecked by pain and disability.

Born in England in 1955 with spina bifida and hydrocephalus, Davis was confined to a wheelchair by the age of fourteen; by thirty,

having developed emphysema, osteoporosis, and arthritis as well, she attempted suicide. At first furious that she survived, she eventually went on to experience a conversion, a pilgrimage to Lourdes, and then twenty-eight years of service to the least and the lost, serving death row inmates in Texas and founding a charity for disabled children in India.

Such a life shows that dignity – a term much bandied about, but which comes from the Latin *dignitas* and means "virtue, worthiness, or honor" – does not depend on autonomy or independence, and certainly not on lack of suffering, but rather on our ability to accept the crosses laid on us in life, and to wait patiently for God's hour when it comes to death.

None of us wants to suffer needlessly. But neither can we ever avoid pain and suffering completely. The very Son of God himself had to endure the bitter agony of the cross, and it was through this ordeal that the world was redeemed. Can we presume to escape with anything less? Alice von Hildebrand says that when we look at suffering in this way, it becomes a privilege: we suffer alongside the Savior. "Be faithful until death," he urges us, "and I will give you the crown of life" (Rev. 2:10).

Absent a living faith, and without the surrounding love of an active community, it is entirely understandable that people want to take death back into their own hands. But as followers of Christ who have been charged with preaching the Good News to all people – who know that there is, to quote the apostle Paul, a "far better way" – we know that those hands are empty, and so we cannot stand silently by.

> Dignity does not depend on autonomy or independence.

Christ the Physician

AUGUSTINE OF HIPPO

You know that our Lord and Savior Jesus Christ is the physician of our eternal health, and that to this end he took the weakness of our nature, that our weakness might not last forever. For he assumed a mortal body, wherein to kill death. And though he was crucified through weakness, as the apostle says, yet he lives by the power of God. They are the words too of the same apostle: "He dies no more, and death shall have no more dominion over him."

These things, I say, are well known to your faith. And there is also this which follows from it: that we should know that all the miracles which he did on the body avail to our instruction, that we may from them perceive that which is not to pass away, nor to have any end. He restored to the blind those eyes which death was sure sometime to close; he raised Lazarus to life who was to die again. And whatever he did for the health of bodies, he did it not that they should be forever; whereas at the last he will give eternal health even to the body itself. But because those things which were not seen, were not believed; by means of these temporal things which were seen, he built up faith in those things which were not seen.

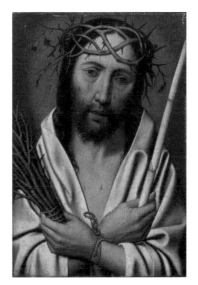

Jan Mostaert,
Christ, Man of Sorrows

Image from Wikimedia Commons (public domain)

These things, then, the Lord did to invite us to the faith. This faith reigns now in the church, which is spread throughout the whole world. And now he works greater cures, on account of which he did not disdain to exhibit those lesser ones.

The physician gave us precepts when we were whole, that we might not need a physician. They that are whole, he says, need not a physician, but they that are sick. When whole we despised these precepts, and by experience have felt how to our own destruction we despised his precepts. Now we are sick, we are in distress, we are on the bed of weakness, yet let us not despair. For because we could not come to the physician, he has vouchsafed to come to us himself.

Come. His house is not too narrow for you; the kingdom of God is possessed equally by all and wholly by each one; it is not diminished by the increasing number of those who possess it, because it is not divided. And that which is possessed by many with one heart is whole and entire for each one. ⌇

Source: Augustine of Hippo, "Sermon 38 on the New Testament," *Nicene and Post-Nicene Fathers, First Series, Vol. 6*, ed. Philip Schaff, trans. R. G. MacMullen (T & T Clark, 1980).

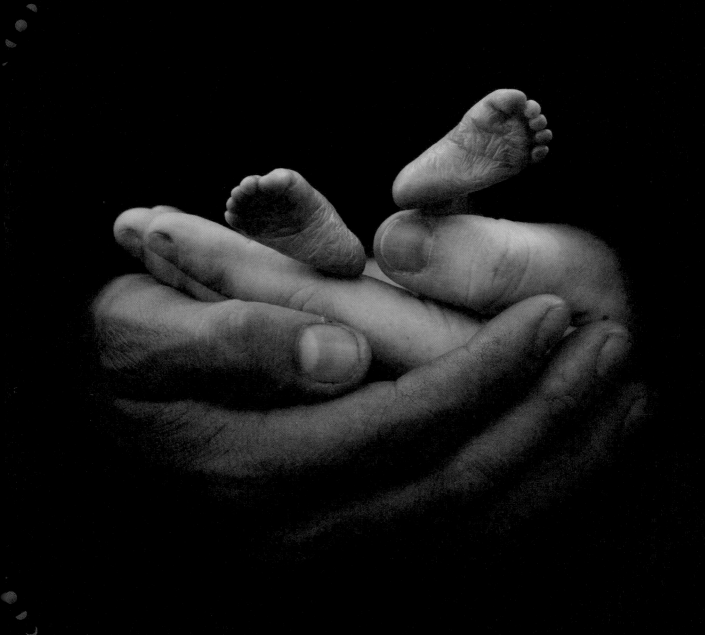

Perfectly Human

*What My Daughter
Taught Me about Beauty,
Worth, and the Gift of Being*

SARAH C. WILLIAMS

Photograph on previous page by Kyle Hartsock. Used by permission.

*t*he doctor's cheery voice gave way to a clipped monotone. He left the room and returned with a female technician. I assumed he was simply inexperienced at doing ultrasounds and bristled with irritation as the woman redid everything he had just done. Then the woman put her hand on my arm and said the words that every expectant mother hopes she will never hear: "I am so sorry, there is something wrong with the baby. We need to fetch the consultant."

"But there can't be," I responded immediately. "I saw the face. The baby looks fine to me." She shook her head and squeezed my arm. I went cold all over.

The consultant sat down beside me. Using the cursor and his finger for reinforcement, he highlighted different points of the tiny person inside me and murmured incomprehensible numbers. "I have to tell you, Mrs. Williams, this baby will not live. It has thanatophoric dysplasia, a lethal skeletal deformity that will certainly result in death shortly after birth. The chest is too small to sustain the proper development of the lungs." A pause. "I suggest you come back with your partner in the morning and we will talk further about what you want to do." A few minutes later I found myself in a side room with a second consultant. Only now did I understand what was meant by the phrase "what you want to do." I listened while the doctor suggested dates for a termination.

"It's the kindest thing to do, isn't it?" I said to Paul that night after our two older daughters were in bed. Once I would have been quick to register my opposition to abortion. Now I was shocked to find that the only thing I wanted was to get the fetus out of my body as quickly as possible. We knew that a stark ethical principle was not enough to carry us through the rest of the pregnancy without hope; it was not enough to enable us to cope with the chance of watching our baby die in pain. Paul suggested we pray.

I can only say we both felt God speak a message to our hearts as clearly as if he had been talking with us in person: *Here is a sick and dying child. Will you love this child for me?* The question reframed everything. It was no longer primarily a question of abstract ethical principle but rather the gentle imperative of love. Before we finished praying, the chasm between the principle and the choice had been filled. As I lay down in my bed that night I realized the decision had been made.

What I did not anticipate in making this decision was the anger that it would provoke in some. One university medic presented the moral arguments in favor of abortion in a robust fashion: "To fail to abort in the case of proven fetal abnormality is morally wrong because in doing so one is deliberately bringing avoidable suffering into the world. It is an ethical imperative to abort in the case of suboptimal life."

I felt like an undergraduate chastised for a weak line of argument in a badly written essay. I knew his words were not intended rudely

---

Dr. Sarah C. Williams has taught history at Oxford and Regent College. She lives with her husband, Paul, in Burford, England. Plough will be releasing her book Perfectly Human: Nine Months with Cerian *in October 2018. Learn more at* plough.com/perfectlyhuman.

or personally – they never are at Oxford – and although I tried only to muse on his argument with the distance of theory, it still kept me awake at night. I knew there was something wrong with his claim. But I could not, as yet, find a defense, and the force of my colleague's case led me to consider whether I was, in fact, being selfish in prolonging the baby's life. The word "suboptimal" rang in my head for days afterwards.

Silently, I formed a counterargument. My medical colleague's argument, along with all the practices I had been pondering, presupposes a particular definition of normality, of health, and of quality of life. But what happens if the definition on which this argument rests is dubious? Whose definition of normality is it anyway? And on what basis is quality of life assessed? What is a normal person? Do normal people have a certain intelligence or skin color? Normality is a relative scale with no accepted criteria in all cultures. At one end of this relative scale we place people who are restricted by intellectual functioning, illness, age, or accident. And at the other end of this scale we place people with efficient minds and bodies. By this definition each of my three children sit at different points on the normality spectrum. Could I as a parent who loves them equally decide which one of them was most valuable, or worthy of a place on the planet?

And what happens if you can't choose, if you can't make decisions for yourself, if you're stripped of agency unexpectedly, through illness or disability? Does this make you a sub-person or a non-person? Are you a pre-person before you achieve anything? And if you are born with no talents and you cannot achieve the proper formation of the body in the womb, does this mean you are not a person?

We named our third daughter Cerian, Welsh for "loved one." Cerian's life ended in the hour before she was born. At that moment the presence of God came powerfully into the hospital room. It was unlike anything I have ever experienced, before or since. Weighty, intimate, holy, the room was full of God. Everything inside me stilled; I hardly dared breathe. His presence was urgent and immediate and I knew with certainty that God

When I made the decision to carry Cerian to term, it felt like the destruction of my plans and hopes.

had come in his love to take a tiny deformed baby home to be with him. There would be no painful bone crushing for Cerian, only the peaceful wonder of God's enfolding presence.

When I first found out about Cerian's deformity and made the choice to carry her to term, it felt like the destruction of my plans and hopes. It went against what I wanted. It limited me. But it was in this place of limitation that God showed me more of his love. Up until this point, the clamor of my desires and wishes had made me like a closed system centered in on myself, on my needs, flaws, and attributes. My life, even at times my religion, had revolved around achievement, reputation, and winning respect and approval from others. I had busied myself with perfect home, perfect children, perfect job, all the things I wanted. I knew I had lost something deep and precious, but I didn't know what it was. And the more I felt the lack of it, the harder I tried to find it through effort. During the nine months I carried Cerian, God came close to me again unexpectedly, wild and beautiful, good and gracious. I touched his presence as I carried Cerian and as a result I realized that underneath all my other longings lay an aching desire for God himself and for his love. Cerian shamed my strength, and in her weakness and vulnerability, she showed me a way of intimacy. The beauty and completeness of her personhood nullified the value system to which I had subscribed for so long.

*t*hree years after Cerian died I was invited to address an international medical conference convened to discuss the effects of prenatal testing policies on women in Western and non-Western contexts. For three hours I was bombarded with questions. It was clear that my views on prenatal testing were of incidental importance to the group; their interest centered on my experience as a mother finding herself in a situation of having to decide suddenly whether or not to terminate a pregnancy. My story exemplified the stark reality that prenatal screening places some parents in the position of *having* to decide the fate of their unborn children, not merely having the *option* to do so.

"What did it feel like to be placed in this position?" All the questions came down to this one in the end. This "necessity to choose," hard though it may be for Western women used to making decisions about their own bodies, is even harder for women in parts of the Middle East, Africa, and South America. Where in a Western context the identification of male and female is in most cases a benign advantage enabling parents to name the little person they are about to welcome into the world and to furnish a new nursery accordingly, in some non-Western contexts revealing the sex places the unborn child at risk of termination on grounds of gender, and mothers at risk of intolerable pressure to abort females.

The chief concern of everyone around the table was to understand how best to *support* women who found themselves in this invidious position. But no one asked whether this *need* to decide was a legitimate or bearable weight for parents, and especially women, to carry? No one disputed the wisdom of implementing prenatal screening programs to detect and diagnose fetal abnormalities.

As I listened to the stories of women from other parts of the world, the ordinary and routine custom of prenatal scanning that we take for granted in the West suddenly became strange to me as I saw it through fresh eyes. Built into the practice is a particular way of perceiving personhood, of defining autonomy and choice, of imagining female agency, of understanding and experiencing community, and of forming identity. The practice relies above all on a particular idea of choice and a definition of personhood in which the capacity for choice is of primary importance. Prenatal scans, though advised, are voluntary – they are customary rather than required – but it is expected nonetheless that most pregnant couples will choose to have one. The practice itself is understood to be morally neutral. It is the degree to which it supports and facilitates individual choice that determines whether or not it is good or bad, right or wrong.

As I listened to the debate going on around me, I remembered the details of Cerian's small, unlovely body. Technically speaking, during the pregnancy there were only two things we knew about her for certain – two scientifically derived facts: the fact of her physical abnormality, and the fact of her biological sex. I wondered if it really is an advantage for these two particular facts to be the first things parents come to know about their children.

What are the implications of this prior knowledge for human society?

Often couples wait to commit emotionally to their unborn child until the "viability" of a pregnancy is confirmed by means of a scan at sixteen or twenty weeks. I hear so many couples say, "We haven't told anyone yet; we're waiting until we've had the scan." They speak as if the scan determines whether or not the pregnancy is real, at least in a social sense; they speak as if the scan were a marker point determining whether they can lavish their love upon the child or hold it back to protect themselves. As a practice, prenatal scanning both teaches and reinforces particular ways of thinking about the human person. It teaches the pregnant couple to ask: Is this child physically normal? This question is asked as if it were of primary importance. Whether or not the scan results reveal fetal abnormality, irrespective of whether a parent chooses to act in certain ways as a result of the information given, the practice makes everyone ask this question at a relatively early stage in the pregnancy. It may only be a tiny statistical minority of parents who choose with much grief and heartache to terminate a pregnancy because of fetal abnormality (and such parents should never be judged). But the fact that we have an almost universal social practice that renders acceptable the *idea* of terminating the life of a child whose physical capacities are suboptimal affects every one of us. This idea is further reinforced by a legal structure that makes such an idea not only plausible but also permissible and possible right up to full term. Moreover, we have sophisticated language to cloak the idea in moral neutrality, and we have a definition of "quality of life" to explain why such an idea is right and necessary.

But do we ever ask whether this idea is *just*? Is it just for the majority of people to condone a social practice that permits a few to be treated in ways the majority would never permit for themselves? Would the majority of people want to be asked, before they were treated with equal dignity and respect, if they have a normal body, or if they are female? To condone this treatment for some not only dehumanizes those who are never born, it dehumanizes all of us. To make human personhood contingent in any way upon physical "normality" is to strip all of us of our inherent and intrinsic worth as persons.

Over the years I have reflected deeply on the weeks and months I spent with Cerian. That period of time felt like an age when I was in the midst of it, but in the scheme of things it was so short. I cannot help but think how easily I might have missed the beauty and the privilege of that time with her. This time of limitation and vulnerability was also a time of profound humanity during which I discovered my need of God, but also my need of others, and their need of me. For nine months every human being has the one chance he or she will ever have of being received first and foremost as a person – before anything else is known

Would the majority of people want to be asked if they have a normal body before they were treated with dignity and respect?

about them. At a time when so many young people struggle intensely with their physicality, with their male or female bodies, with their identities as sexual beings, with the health and appearance of their body, the nine months of pregnancy may be the only opportunity we will have as parents to receive our child simply as a person of equal, inviolable worth whether the child turns out to be healthy or sick, male or female, attractive or plain. Why are we choosing to rob ourselves of this extraordinary and unique gift?

Precious though we all understand children to be, we behave as if they were commodities – commodities that we acquire as an extension of ourselves. We have grown familiar with the idea of conferring personhood selectively on the ones we choose because we find them desirable, preferable, and acceptable. Indeed, in the Western world, choosing what we desire has become the essence of what it means to be human.

Our society tells us that our choices are unlimited, that choice is the means to human flourishing, that to have one's choices impaired is to be dehumanized. As a society we try to deal with suffering by controlling it, mastering it, and seeking to eliminate it. If we fail in this endeavor then at least we hide it, we silence the

> *God the creator came in his love to take a vulnerable human being home to be with him.*

mention of it, we insure heavily against it, we insulate ourselves from it, we resolve to ignore it. We mask the reality of death.

And yet this idea of humanness defined by choice, into which we are all baptized, does not line up with our messy, complicated, everyday humanness. It has nothing to say when aging creeps into our bones, wrinkles our skin, reduces our eyesight, and limits our energy. It has no dignity to give us when we become dependent on others, and no dignity to give

to those who care for others. It has no time beyond the moment, and no validity beyond experience. It does not prepare us for the powerlessness that comes to all of us when our choices fail, when the scope of choice narrows, when our choices are overlooked, violated, or curtailed by others. We find ourselves trapped in the contradictions of the world we have created for ourselves.

*a*gainst this backdrop, the quiet beauty of Cerian's life goes on challenging me: *What does it really mean to be human?* Cerian didn't have any choices, and yet she was perfectly human.

The overriding memory of my time with Cerian, the one I will carry with me for the rest of my life, was the glimpse I had, during the moments of her death, of the love and glory of God. That memory causes all the other recollections, good and bad, to pale in comparison. God the creator came in his love to take a vulnerable human being home to be with him. This encounter changed my life. Quite simply, it showed me that there is another way to be in the world.

Limitation, finitude, suffering, weakness, disability, and frailty can be gifts. Far from robbing us of our humanity, these things are needed if we are to be human. Without them, we strip ourselves of the opportunity to confer dignity on each other regardless of our physical and mental condition and we lose sight of the essential given-ness of human life. Ultimately, personhood is not a work of self-definition and self-creation. Instead, it is a gift. ⤝

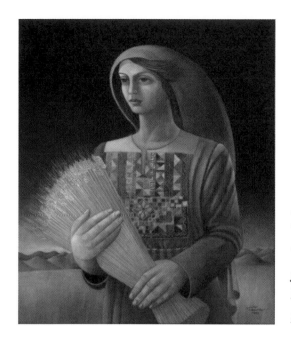

Hold On

When you reap the harvest of your land, do not . . .
gather the gleanings of your harvest. . . .
Leave them for the poor and the foreigner.
Leviticus 19:9–10

This grip of patience, after the scythe
cuts in. Most have dropped – relieved –
into gathering arms – brusque, adequate,
but this foolish remnant holds their roots.

Perhaps they have made this calculation:
on the one hand, to become a clean-scrubbed
loaf on the landowner's table, surrounded
by his ruddy children and their stout grins.

On the other to be plucked by a strange
or timid hand, rolled right there for all
to start at their plump kernels shed
by unfluent palms, and the perfect snap

of a willing seed between hungry teeth.
For the meek inherit a happy earth.

SUZANNE   HARLAN   HEYD

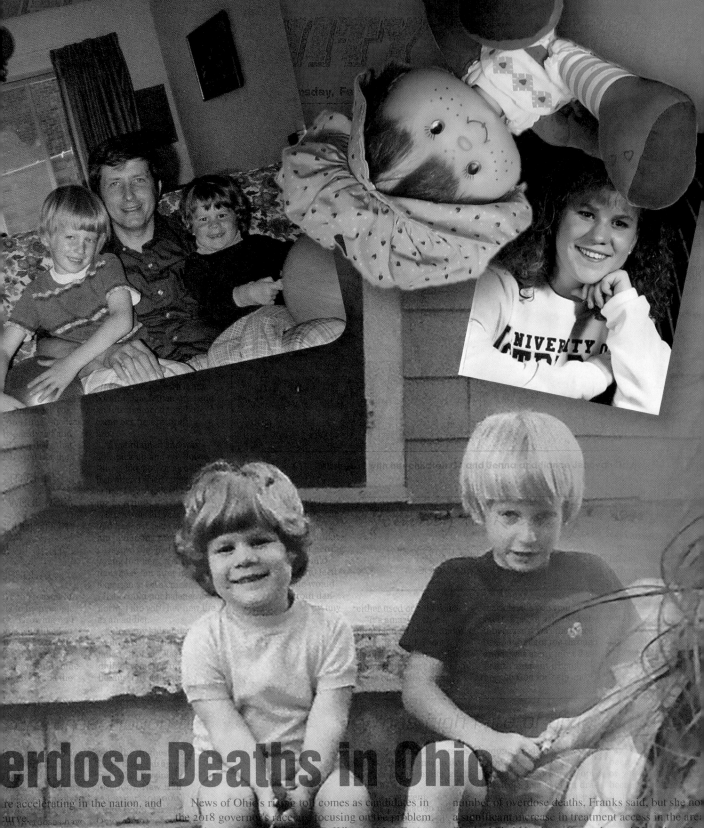

erdose Deaths in Ohio

re accelerating in the nation, and
urve.
tate rank 2nd in the number of
ehind only West Virginia, the
uing and possibly accelerating in
w.
aid Nan Franks, CEO of Addic
a nonprofit that is at the forefront
epidemic in Greater Cincinnati
ky.
for Health Statistics report
nal overdose death counts from

News of Ohio's rising toll comes as candidates in
the 2018 governor's race are focusing on the problem.
Both Attorney General Mike DeWine and Lt. Gov.
Mary Taylor are making how they would tackle the
opioid crisis a key part of their campaigns.

The Cincinnati area, including Northern Kentucky,
has been fighting the opioid epidemic with cooperation
from multiple levels of health, government, nonprofit,
social services and law enforcement, Franks said. But
she knows more needs to be done.

"We will need to commit more resources, more
funding, to continue to make progress," she said.

number of overdose deaths, Franks said, but she no
a significant increase in treatment access in the are.
She included Northern Kentucky and Hamilton Cou
as areas adding intensive outpatient services, and n
that there's more treatment available outside the co
such as the Northland Treatment Center in Clermor
County.

Wandersleben said that the use of medication-
assisted treatment, or "MAT," the best evidence-ba
treatment for heroin or other opioid addiction, is
growing in Ohio. "In April, about 50,000 people in
Ohio were receiving MAT. As of this month, it has

Let Me Stand

My sister died of an overdose.
But first, she forgave me.

MARK SCHLONEGER

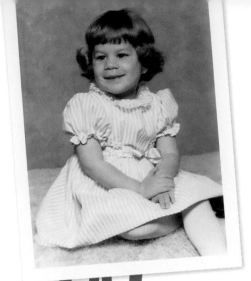

Tricia at age three

Photographs courtesy of the author

When my sister Tricia was three years old, Heather pushed her down. Heather, who lived in a neighboring house and was Tricia's age, had been talking with her on the front stoop when the two girls had a difference of opinion. But it ended with a push from Heather, and Tricia on the ground.

Most young children would have forgotten the incident almost immediately. But not Tricia. To her, that push was an injustice that could not stand. "Heather pushed me down," she proclaimed to Dad and Mom. "Heather pushed me down," she informed me that night from the lower bunk. "Heather pushed me down," she announced to aunts, uncles, grandmas, grandpas, and every subsequent visitor to our home. Several months later, when we moved to Ohio, she was still repeating the line to a whole new audience.

Last year, grieving my sister's death, I remembered the Heather Incident and wept. That's because Heather turned out to be a recurring character in Tricia's life story. "Heather pushed me down" was a three-year-old's cry for justice, a tiny fist raised in defiance against the powers conspiring against her. Over and over and over, Tricia announced to the world what had happened to her and who had done it. Then, she stopped.

Sometimes, the Heathers she faced were people taking advantage of a vulnerable girl. Sometimes they were the result of her own choices. No matter their origin, Tricia's Heathers kept pushing, pushing, pushing. At some point, she stopped believing it was an injustice worthy of protest. Maybe she simply accepted it, even came to expect it. As she grew older, I think she learned what the world seemed to be teaching her: "You deserve it."

While the first three years of my life were spent in a protective, loving home, Tricia's experience in her birth and foster homes must have been on earth as it is in hell. She struggled her entire life to find healing from the abuse she experienced as a baby and toddler. And, if she ever thought she could forget it, her body was there to remind her.

Whenever she looked in the mirror, cigarette burn scars appeared for her reflection. Whenever she touched her left wrist, another scar marked the hump it once carried, the broken bone that had gone untreated. Cosmetics and surgery hid the blemish, straightened the bone, and never touched the wound.

Until Tricia came into our family, I was the youngest of three boys. Suddenly, I was a new big brother, delighted to move up to the top bunk. Having a girl in the family meant I had to dig through endless Strawberry Shortcake accessories to get to my Hot Wheels in the family toy box. It was always Strawberry Shortcake for Tricia – they shared the same dazzling red hair.

On the evening of her first day in our family, we all ate popcorn and watched *The Wizard of Oz* on television. I was terrified by the flying monkeys and couldn't finish the movie, but three-year-old Tricia stayed to the end, captivated. From that day and through all the years ahead, she watched *The Wizard of Oz* whenever it was on. We didn't know, that first time, how much her life would resemble a lost girl on a strange road, looking for a way back.

In elementary school, a learning disability limited her progress and magnified her limitations. In middle school, she was raped by a boy a few years older than her, a family acquaintance. He threatened to kill her if she told anyone. She didn't, until a few years ago. "Heather pushed me down?" That was for three-year-olds. Now, she raged against my parents, my brothers, and me. At night, I began locking my bedroom door.

In high school, I heard someone in the lunch line talking about Tricia. She was easy, he said. She put out. She was a slut.

I was enraged and embarrassed. I wanted to punch him, to push his head against the wall, to make him bleed. But I did nothing, said nothing.

As an adult, Tricia was unable to give and receive love in a consistent way. She struggled with multiple addictions and was often jailed for drug-related offenses. She was regularly unemployed because she was regularly undependable. Her relationships with family members were often strained. She loved her two children deeply, but wasn't able to mother them as she wanted and as they deserved. In her pain, she inflicted pain on others – and accepted the pain inflicted by others.

Then came the day when a doctor addressed Tricia's complaints of chronic pain with an opioid prescription. When the prescription ran out, she turned to heroin. It was heroin that took over her life before taking her life.

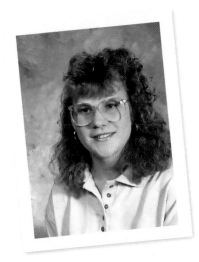

Tricia in high school

One weekend in November, 2016, the small town of Wooster, Ohio, reported six heroin overdoses. The Channel 5 Evening News reported:

> Like many Northeast Ohio cities, Wooster has seen an increase in the number of suspected heroin overdoses in recent months. But police say they've never seen anything like the surge that happened Thursday between 3 and 11 p.m. Wooster police chief Matt Fisher said two of the overdoses left people on life support. . . . "Listen, they're somebody's son," said Fisher. "They're somebody's daughter, aunt, niece, nephew. There's people that love them."

Mark Schloneger is pastor of North Goshen Mennonite Church and lives in Goshen, Indiana, with his wife and three children.

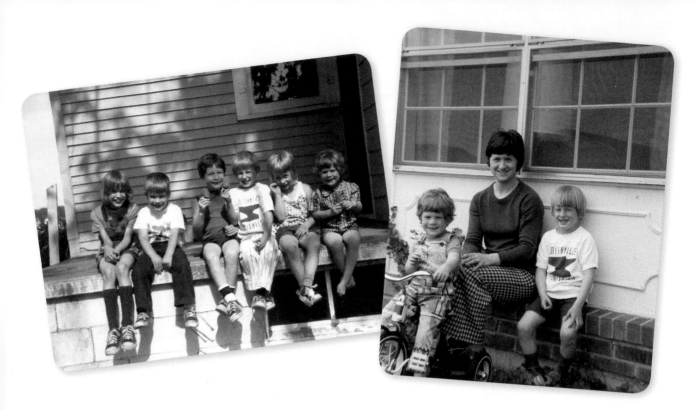

This report garnered its share of Facebook comments, including someone's attempted witticism, modified from a popular meme: "I'm not saying they deserve to die, but I'd unplug their life-support to charge my cell phone."

Two people died that weekend. One of them was my sister. She was worth more than a cell phone.

The heroin epidemic in our towns and cities is nothing short of demonic. Heroin and other drugs gain a foothold in vulnerable people and then demand more space. They cause people to hurt themselves and to push away those who love them the most. They distort people's images so they can't be who they were created to be. They enter, coerce, possess, then kill. Do I believe in demons? You don't doubt their existence when they're on your doorstep, pushing.

But they are elsewhere too. There's a spirit of evil alive in the callousness of those who have not been thrown down by addiction, who lightly post, as in another response to an overdose report: "Let them die. If they can afford [to] do the drugs. . . . We all have choices in life."

Yes, choices. Sometimes those choices are options like Fall and Fall Again. During Tricia's last stint in jail, she wrote out her statement to the judge before her sentencing hearing: "I am forty-three years old, and I've had a lifetime of bad choices and decisions that have caused much destruction to all of those who love me. And I am done. I don't want to live like this any longer. I just don't have much fight and survival left in me. I want to truly have a chance at a normal, healthy life." She described her plans to join a women's support group because she "no longer wants to live under the influence of heroin and everything else that goes along [with it]."

"With prayer and God's grace," she wrote, "I will take one day and one step at a time."

The jail chaplain and others who visited her vouched for her sincerity. They said that she truly wanted to make changes in her life, that she acknowledged her addiction and made plans to get an injection to help manage its power. They said that they liked her. I wasn't surprised. In her later years, she was most truly herself when she was in jail: funny, charming, generous, and genuine.

Tricia was released from the Wayne County Jail on Thursday, November 3, 2016. Hours after her release, a friend and former supplier searched for her like a twisted shepherd looking for one lost sheep. He found her at her daughter's apartment and then led her to the valley of death. This time, the heroin was laced with fentanyl. For the final time, Heather pushed Tricia down. She never got back up.

When I was around ten years old, I had a dream that shook me from sleep. It was one of those dreams that won't fade in the morning sun. To this day, I remember it vividly. Tricia is chasing me. I sprint down streets, dart through yards, cut across fields, but I can't escape her. I rush up the steps to a large house and stop to open the door. When Tricia comes up behind me, I spin around and push her with all of my strength. She tumbles backwards off the porch and down the steps, and lies still on the sidewalk below. When I go to look more closely, it's not Tricia on the sidewalk. It's the baby Jesus, looking up at me.

For many years, this dream tormented me. Throughout my life, I've been angry at Tricia as well as ashamed by her, afraid of her, and worried for her. I've been angry at God as I prayed for Tricia. I've been angry – am still angry – at those who abused her, used her, raped her, and discarded her. But my most consistent feeling concerning Tricia was guilt, a feeling that my dream seemed to reinforce.

With time, I came to understand how my desperate need to achieve, to earn approval, stemmed from a desire to prove to others that I was not like my sister. For a troubled girl seeking affirmation, how hard it must have been to have a brother determined to grasp the very things that would never be in her reach. For an exploited girl seeking solace, how hard it must have been to have a brother on a mission to prove that his sister was not his parents' fault. For a vulnerable girl seeking safety, how hard it must have been to have a brother who wouldn't speak and act in her defense. The truth is, I was one of Tricia's Heathers.

Several years ago, I felt convicted to ask Tricia for forgiveness. She was in jail at the time. By appearances, I was a successful brother – a pastor – generously leaving his loving family to visit his failure sister – a felon – languishing again behind bars. In reality, our positions were reversed. She held all of the power, and I was afraid. I had no idea how she might respond. I knew she couldn't run away – she was in jail, after all – but we had never really talked on a deep level about anything, much less about how we had hurt each other. I didn't know how she thought of these things, or if she ever did.

The guard unlocked, then re-locked, door after door. He ushered me into a bleak, block-walled room, and I sat down on a lopsided folding chair. When Tricia came in, she was happy, excited to see me, as always. We talked as we always did. She asked about my wife, Sarah, and each of our children. When I asked how things had been for her recently, she began evaluating area jails as if she were writing Yelp reviews. We laughed together, and I was tempted to leave with the good feeling of a good conversation during a good visit.

But then, with an aching lump in my throat, I choked into words the reason for my visit, spanning several decades of guilt. She listened as I asked for mercy. And then, she forgave me – immediately, completely, without minimizing my need. My sister, my confessor, granted me the absolution that she never fully knew.

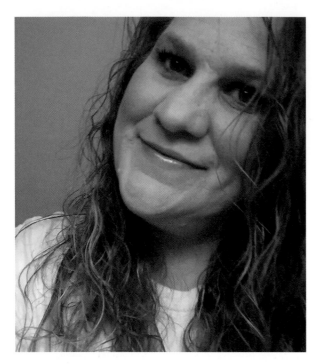

Tricia, 2014

After Tricia died, my thoughts returned to that vivid dream. It had haunted so many of my waking hours; now it became a comfort in my grieving ones. Lying on that sidewalk, pushed down by me and untold others, the Christ Child lies where my sister fell.

Tricia faced many Heathers in her life. Some were of her own creation, but others were people like me, broken people inflicting pain from a place of pain. In the end, the distinction does not matter. Are any of our choices made in complete isolation from the choices of others, for good or for ill? Can anyone be solely responsible for his or her successes or failures? Wouldn't it be more truthful to acknowledge that people cannot solely navigate their lives as either helpless victims or solitary warriors?

In the end, these sorts of philosophical questions are asked only by people who are standing. Once you've fallen, it doesn't matter how you got there. You just want to get up. You long for someone to help you, to take you by the hand, to lift you up, and to walk with you so that you won't fall again.

When Tricia's funeral service was over, everyone walked across the parking lot to share a meal in the church fellowship hall. That's when Stacy, one of Tricia's friends, waved me over and asked me where she could go for a smoke. Being at church, she didn't want people to see her. I directed her to a place just around the corner, but she asked if I could go with her to show her.

My heart sank. I was physically and emotionally spent, and all I wanted to do was claim a seat with family members who I hadn't seen in far too long. I had walked with Stacy only a few more steps when she stopped, lit up a cigarette, and told me to stay in front of her. She gave me no choice. I was her human shield against the condemnation she expected and the shame she felt. So she smoked, and I stood. And the more she smoked and the more I stood, the more I thought that this was the perfect way to remember my sister. With smoke on my clothes, I gave thanks to God for Tricia – deeply flawed, deeply human, deeply loved, and deeply loving. Only God knows how many times we fall. Only God knows how many times no one is there to pick us up. But this I believe: the living Christ waits in the places where we fall. Together, my sister, we rise. ⤳

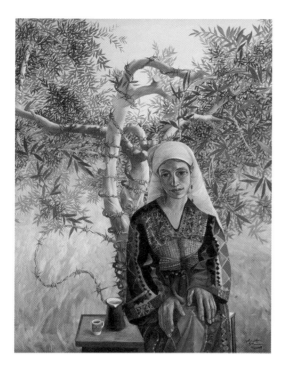

Suleiman Mansour,
Quiet Morning

To Sing

By the rivers of Babylon we sat and wept
when we remembered Zion.
There on the poplars we hung our harps,
for there our captors asked us for songs . . . of joy.
Psalm 137:1–3

Every harp hung on a poplar
left a mute slew of fingers.

There was still the bread-making, the
laundry, the struggle with the tongue-
twisted rope of the well. Later infernal
socks to darn; still later typewriter keys.

Those, of all, came close to singing.

But even now, if you hold out your hands –
nails up – you will see them tremble,
ever so slightly. Like a tuning fork or
vibratoed note, remembering, trying.

SUZANNE HARLAN HEYD

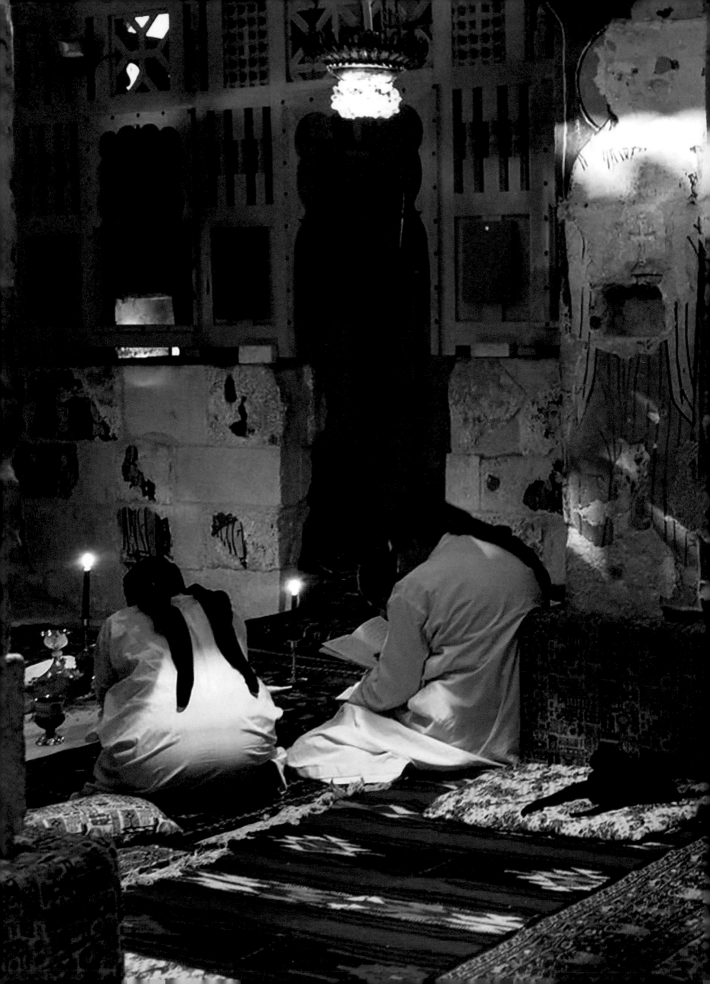

Photography
by Cécile Massie

All Sorts of Little Things

ON COMPASSION IN A TIME OF WAR

— STEPHANIE SALDAÑA —

The image is remarkable. On Good Friday, photographer Cécile Massie was sitting in the chapel at the monastery of Deir Mar Musa in the heart of Syria, observing the monastic community at prayer, when a young Muslim visitor slipped in, carrying his prayer rug. He sought out a discreet corner of the chapel, turned towards Mecca, and began to pray.

Cécile snapped a photo [*previous spread*]. So it is that the rest of us can now peer into this moment of intimacy, carried out in a country seven years into war, of a Muslim and Christians praying in a remote church together, each in their own tradition – a moment that might have otherwise been lost to history and witnessed only by God.

I have returned to that photograph repeatedly in the last weeks – as though that shared prayer might somehow hold the fractured world in place. In time, details have emerged: the wooden figure of Christ, removed from the cross after Good Friday services and placed on the ground in preparation for burial, is just visible on the furthest left corner of the photo, illuminated by candlelight. The icons on the iconostasis have been turned inward for mourning.

In the dimness of the chapel, the photo is made possible by light coming in from an open door. Together and separately the Muslim and Christian faithful turn toward God. This shared prayer – and with it a hope – enters into our suffering and becomes known.

The word *compassion,* in its most basic form, means to "suffer with," or, to "share the suffering" of another. But in watching them I am reminded of another word

that has the same root – Christ's *Passion,* that ultimate gesture of shared suffering for the sake of love. For Christians, perhaps compassion in a time of war might best be thought of as a "sharing of the Passion," a recognition that we cannot love one another if we shield ourselves from the hardships our neighbors have endured. The monks and nuns of Deir Mar Musa, a Christian monastic community dedicated to dialogue with Islam, only exist in the photo at all because they, at great risk to their lives, decided to remain in Syria throughout the war. Father Jacques Mourad, a Syrian priest and member of the community, wrote about the renewed significance of wartime dialogue in a letter in 2014, quoted by Navid Kermani in the pages of this magazine [Spring 2016]: "Right now, the kind of dialogue we're experiencing is our shared suffering as a community. We are sorrowing in this unjust world, which bears a share of the responsibility for the victims of the war, this world of the dollar and the euro, which cares only for its own citizens, its own wealth, and its own safety while the rest of the world dies of hunger, sickness, and war. . . . The true dialogue we are living today is the dialogue of compassion."

Since then, the world has continued to look on as Syrian innocents have been shot or crushed, gassed or drowned, downed by easily preventable illnesses, and left to die in too many ways to mention here. Many of us who live in the region are tempted to despair. The numbers of the dead have likely climbed to over 500,000 – an estimated 2.3 percent of the region's pre-war population. UN agencies have stopped counting. Those who are killed no longer have names, nor

Photographs reproduced by permission of Cécile Massie

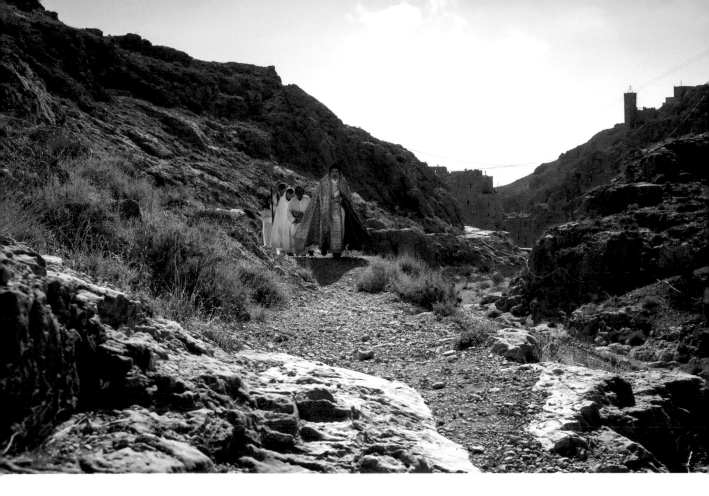

numbers – they seem not to matter at all. And those suffering today are hardly confined to Syria: I recently saw thousands waiting in squalid conditions in a Greek refugee and migrant camp who had fled Iraq, Iran, Afghanistan, Yemen, and the Democratic Republic of Congo, among other countries: only some of the estimated 65.6 million individuals displaced worldwide. Those not fleeing war were fleeing poverty. The scale was astonishing.

Here in Jerusalem, where I live, many predict that a new wave of violence will also erupt soon. Already we wait on Fridays for news of Palestinian protestors killed and wounded by the hundreds in Gaza, and then we return to our daily affairs. I fear that most of us – myself included – have become used to this violence. We speak of the dead with the same nonchalance we once reserved for the weather, or traffic that might inconvenience us on the way to work. When a priest I know was recently asked about the situation in the region, he answered with shocking honesty: "We are sleepwalking towards disaster."

Is there a way out? I think back to Father Jacques' words. A dialogue of *compassion,* a binding of ourselves together in love, might be all we have left – carried out in a world that no longer cares.

Palm Sunday procession at Deir Mar Musa monastery, 2018

Stephanie Saldaña is a writer based in the Middle East and the author of, most recently, A Country Between. *She lives in Jerusalem with her husband and children.*

Yet if compassion asks all of us to "suffer with," it begs the question: who should we suffer with? To whom should we bind ourselves in this hour of need? If we listen to the prevailing wisdom not only in the Middle East but also abroad, then we should be cautious of who we choose to suffer with – for there is only so much suffering the human heart can bear. How many times have I heard Christian clergy ask the faithful to pray for the "Christians of the Middle East," neglecting to mention that millions of people of other faiths have been killed or uprooted by the current wars? They suggest that we should "suffer with" only those of our own confession. How often have European leaders reminded us that they have *compassion* in principle, but that Europe cannot be asked to take in more migrants? How often have American politicians reminded us that they have *compassion,* but that we would do better not to interfere in the Middle East – even if that only means offering funds for refugees to go to school? Even members of aid agencies have privately told me that they have *compassion,* but that economic migrants are complicating the narrative they wish to tell about offering asylum to victims of war – as if poverty were not a violence that one might need to flee. Yes, of course we are willing to *suffer with* . . . but the question of *who* we suffer with is something else entirely. Yes, I have *compassion!* . . . But I will suffer only with those of my own religion, my own country, my own family, my own social class, my own politics. . . . Never have I heard so many preconditions. People are willing to suffer, but on their own terms.

How tempting it is to give in to this logic of scarcity, repeated so confidently by those in power! One wonders what has happened to the faith of the loaves and fishes. The miracle of the wine. The promise that love does not need to be siphoned off – indeed, that love multiplies.

Who is my neighbor? Who do I suffer with?

We stand at a precipice. I am increasingly convinced that the only way back is to choose to bind ourselves however possible to every person we encounter. I say this not out of some naïve hope, but out of a grim reality, that the alternative is rising nationalism and a brutal sectarianism.

Who will I suffer with? Everyone, without exception. We can only hope to be saved together.

These days, when I am tempted to give up, I often think of Christian de Chergé, the prior of the monastery of Tibhirine, the monastic community of French Cistercian monks who decided to remain in Algeria during the country's civil war so as not to abandon their Muslim neighbors. Seven of the monks, including Christian, eventually lost their lives due to their fidelity. Pope Francis recently recognized them as martyrs, clearing the way for their beatification.

During the period leading up to their deaths, Christian wrote often of the monks' "martyrdom of love" – not their eventual deaths, but their choice to live out – day by day, moment by moment – a solidarity with the suffering of those with whom they shared their daily lives. Remarking that their choice to stay was a choice to live "in constancy" with others who suffered, he placed the brothers in communion with the Muslims with whom they lived, noting that "this place [Algeria] has other inhabitants who are also our brothers in constancy in this difficult time."

He often returned to the example of Christ washing the feet of his disciples before his Passion. In a Holy Thursday sermon, Chergé wrote: "From experience, we know that small gestures cost a lot, especially if they are

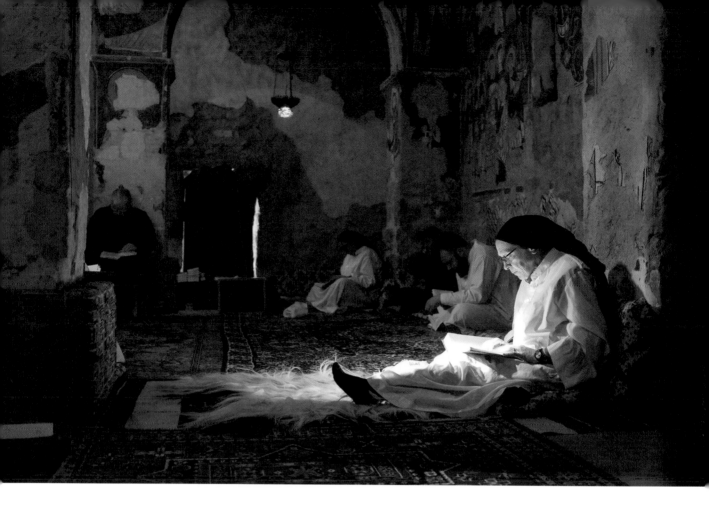

repeated each day. We wash the feet of our brothers on Holy Thursday, but what would it be like to do this daily? And to all who come?" For Chergé, martyrdom of love is accomplished only through "all sorts of little things."

All sorts of little things. What kinds of little things? Might we also learn them?

For when I think about this moment we find ourselves in, it is not the bombed-out cities that frighten me most, the ravaged homes and mosques, churches and town squares – though these losses are devastating. It is the destroyed relationships. In this I fear that all of us have become guilty, be it from the hatred that has built up in our hearts, to the indifference – its own form of violence – that has kept us from caring anymore. We have come to believe the fiction that we can live without one another. There will be no brick and mortar that will repair this, no shortcut that will bring us back again after we have so dehumanized others and in doing so lost much of our own humanity. We will only make our way back day by day, moment by moment, through *all sorts of little things.*

I have witnessed these *little things* carried out by ordinary people, often refugees, who have discovered within their hearts some wellspring of kindness that survived war and displacement. It is in large part because of them that I have not given up yet. I think of a young refugee who fled years of bloodshed in

Morning prayer at the monastery of Deir Mar Musa

Easter Vigil, four a.m. The first text is read in the dark before Mass is celebrated.

Deir ez-Zor in Syria and was stranded on an island in Greece. He sat his friend down in a folding chair outside the camp and lovingly gave him a haircut.

I stood back in awe, witnessing this *little thing*.

Or Sanaa, a Syrian woman I met in Jordan who lost her brother in the war, and who I watched leaning over a kitchen table and helping her son with his homework.

An exhausted Palestinian day laborer who gave up his seat on the bus after a day of work, recognizing that an old man was carrying a heavier burden, still.

A Syrian priest who was kidnapped and escaped, forgiving the one who betrayed him.

A former prisoner who still bore the scars of torture on his body, singing as he prepared a meal for his friends.

A community of monks and nuns, who decided to stay.

How can God possibly be indifferent to such gestures? How can any of us? When we have given up on institutions to save us, on governments or aid agencies, on political leaders, we place our hope in these small, almost invisible acts to repair the world. *Little things* are elevated to their proper place in the story of salvation, as miracles, a dialogue of pots and pans, often carried out by anonymous saints – mothers and fathers and their children, gardeners and bakers – who remind us through their tenderness how to be human again.

Somewhere in a Syrian village, a father plants a tree. A young man crosses the sea with his violin wrapped in cellophane. A Muslim man walks into a Christian chapel in a country at war, turns toward Mecca, and joins the two communities in prayer.

And the world holds out another day, in expectation of almond blossoms, or a symphony. ➤

The Measure of a Life Well Lived

CLARE STOBER

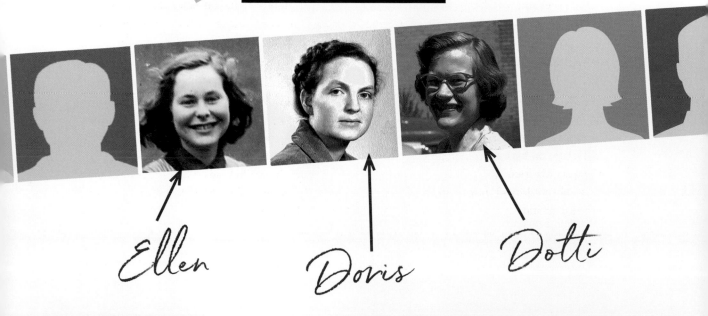

Ellen

Doris

Dotti

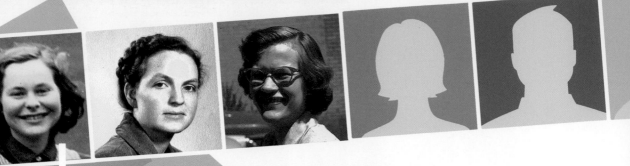

All images courtesy of the families of Ellen Keiderling, Doris Mercer, and Dotti Button. Used with permission.

Just over a year ago, I sat by my father's bed for ten days and nights, watching him die. We connected through touch as I held his weakening hand, swabbed out his mouth, and did all I could to ease his last passage. I stroked his forearms, still so familiar, and recalled everything I'd known about him and done with him, this man who had always been there.

"But what is the measure of a life well lived?" The question, as persistent as it was answerless, kept interrupting – interrogating – the memories that flowed through my mind. After he died I reentered normal life, returning home to the Bruderhof, the Christian community to which I belong, just in time to attend the funeral of an old friend. This loss was quickly followed by two more funerals, for two other old friends. And it seemed, as I remembered their characters and listened to the stories of their lives, that these three women were giving me one last gift, extending an answer to the question that had dogged my vigil at my father's side.

As a boomer growing up in the relative comfort and prosperity of the fifties, I used to assume that every college-educated, middle-class woman of my parents' generation aspired to becoming the perfect housewife, patterning herself on Donna Reed or the fictitious Betty Crocker. When I came to the Bruderhof, however, I discovered dozens of women from the "Greatest Generation" who had traded upwardly-mobile comforts and Sunday Christianity for a life of poverty and discipleship.

These three friends were among them.

Dotti died first, but she was always first – the first to speak, to laugh, to get up and dance (when her legs still worked). A Detroit native, Dotti talked loud, laughed loud, and, well, dressed loud. You could easily pick her out in a crowd by the clownishly bright clothes she wore to keep the ever-lurking depression at bay. She thrived on excitement, hated routine, and felt it her duty to get those around her to live with the same wholehearted purpose.

Perhaps I was drawn to Dotti because she reminded me of my mother. They were the same age, had attended the same art school (missing one another by a year), and were equally high-maintenance. But in Dotti I found an extra depth, a different perspective, a person who'd seen and experienced the same things that had turned my mother into a jaded cynic, but who'd found a way through the darkness to discover joy.

When Dotti said something, you listened. Her sharply worded observations may have sounded off-the-cuff but they came from deep within, a place of wisdom honed by suffering and repentance.

In her twenties, a self-consciously sophisticated art student, Dotti found her life upended in one short weekend in 1952 when she reluctantly attended the Annual Conference of the Women's International League for Peace and Freedom. In her words:

> When I left home on Thursday, I was what I had been brought up to be – a middle

---

Clare Stober is creative director for Plough Publishing House. She lives at Fox Hill, a Bruderhof in Walden, New York.

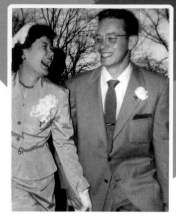

Dotti and Bill →

class, college-educated young lady. When I returned home on Sunday evening, I was a totally different person. My whole attitude toward war, toward minorities, toward poor people, toward unions, toward *everything* was completely changed. The focus of my life after that was to work for world peace, for justice, and for reconciliation between people.

It was her Christian faith that gave context to her new commitment. Dotti and her husband Bill (they married in 1953) were churchgoers. Like the other members of the progressive, integrated Methodist church they attended in Detroit, they focused their faith on social justice and racial reconciliation. In the summer of 1962, intrigued by reports about a pacifist Christian community whose members share all things in common, they decided to go see for themselves. And once again, in the course of a few days, the direction of Dotti's life changed.

Three things they experienced on that first visit to the Bruderhof drew them: the members' obvious joy despite their impoverished circumstances, the fact that people were able to disagree and yet still come to unity, and the outreaching love that Dotti felt from the gathered community. This love was evident in the community celebrations, but it shone through as well as members honestly and openly confronted each other.

In the car on the way back to Detroit Bill announced, "I'm going back." Dotti later recalled:

Bill did not say, "We are going back," or, "Are we going back?" or, "What do you think?" He said, "I am going back." He was called. That is something I have hung on to. No matter what

happens in life, Bill was called to this life by God. I felt the same call, which was more than fortunate: it was God-given. Otherwise, it could have split our family. I had become discouraged, disillusioned, and our marriage was in danger of breaking up. That one weekend turned everything around and gave me a real joy in life.

Ellen died twice. And I am certain that was the key to her joy. But I'm getting ahead of myself.

Ellen would tell you she started out as a "nice Jewish girl from Brooklyn." She was on a search, but for a cause, not – like many of her post-war peers – for the perfect man. Fueled by vague dissatisfaction with the status quo, with a desire for society to be "turned upside down" and for a "solution" to racial injustice, impulsive Ellen set out alone for Europe in 1953 at twenty. One of eleven passengers on a freighter, she spent the five-day voyage holed up in her cabin reading Tolstoy's *War and Peace*.

During that trip, bored with touring London, Ellen decided to "swing by" a Christian community in Shropshire that she'd heard about from a friend in Manhattan. Swinging by entailed multiple train transfers and a fifteen-mile bicycle ride, since the Wheathill Bruderhof was located in the hills near the Welsh border. But when Ellen arrived,

Ellen

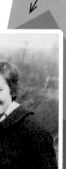

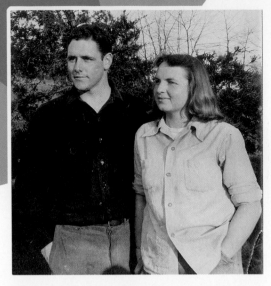

she met far more than she had expected:

> On the way down the driveway I had what I can only call a Damascus Road experience. I looked out over the valley towards Birmingham and had this overwhelming sensation that I was on holy ground, that this place I was standing on had been here from the beginning and would be here forever, into all eternity. This was a call from God. I was Jewish, an atheist, and it was as if God put his hand on my shoulder and said, "You belong here; you have come home." I fell in love with Wheathill from that moment. I never forgot feeling, "This is it. This is home. This is more than home. This is *the* solution."

And so she stayed. At Wheathill, living conditions were bleak – penetrating cold, very little food or warm clothes, no indoor plumbing. Yet Ellen responded with her whole heart when she heard that call. Years later she would write to a grandson: "When I first came to Wheathill I remember going down the driveway and looking out over the view and thinking, 'There must be a God after all.' I always remember the joy that filled me like I had never experienced before. I wanted to sell everything I had and buy the whole field for joy. About finding faith: I think faith finds you."

Doris was the third to die that

spring. Doris, who had grown up as a Quaker in the Finger Lakes region of upstate New York, was Dotti's complete opposite, and was none too similar to Ellen either. Where the other two women seemed to blurt out their feelings without editing, Doris rarely voiced her thoughts. Getting to know her took time

and patience. Small talk got you nowhere. Remaining fully present during what felt like long, full silences was a must.

Although Doris was quiet, she was never self-absorbed. Her greatest pleasures were making crafts from natural materials she'd collected, or sitting outdoors and observing or drawing. Whatever she made, she gave away. Hers was an interior life of reflection and concern for those who didn't "have it all together." Doris was someone you could trust, an oasis of calm and solidity. And so I was surprised to learn, after she passed away, of her own long struggle with feelings of inadequacy and unworthiness.

Doris had experienced something like communal life growing up – her parents taught in a boarding school, where her father was farm manager. She went on to study botany at Cornell. After graduating, she married Bud, who like her had had a taste of intentional community in the Civilian Public Service camp in which he had spent much of World War II as a conscientious objector. After the war, the couple explored a range of communitarian experiments. Then a friend shared with them a letter from a fellow Quaker explaining why he had become a member of the Bruderhof:

> We have for so many years sought for an answer to the causes of the terrible wars, the

inequality and injustice among men that now it is a great joy to throw ourselves completely into this positive effort to demonstrate the possibility of a brotherly way of life.

Bud and Doris went to visit the community a few months later, and soon decided to stay.

Crucibles

Each of these women chose early to live for an ideal, and each gladly gave up her personal freedom and the conventional ingredients of the good life to live a life of meaning and purpose when they joined the community. But not one of them, after making this commitment, "lived happily ever after." It doesn't work that way.

Each of them endured physical, mental, or emotional suffering that put their faith, and their commitment, to the test. That is where each of them found an all-powerful love that sustained them and gave them a purpose to endure their darkest hours. Each, in her own way and words, would have told you she encountered this love in the person of Jesus. "It is a terrible thing to fall into the hands of the living God," Dorothy Day, the founder of the Catholic Worker movement, once wrote. "It is not anything that we can take except with the utmost seriousness and yet it is of course the greatest joy in the world."

In 1967, just five years after Dotti and her family had come to the Bruderhof, her husband Bill abruptly left. The reasons were complicated – decades later, Bill would simply say that he'd had a "heartless mind and a lot of stubborn pride." He'd fully intended to take his wife and children with him, but Dotti refused to go. Instead, she stayed true to the conviction that they'd been called to follow God in community. Over the next five years she single-handedly raised their six children (ranging in age from three months to fifteen when he left), never knowing if Bill would return.

It was like a miracle when he finally did.

*Bill
and
Dotti
and kids*

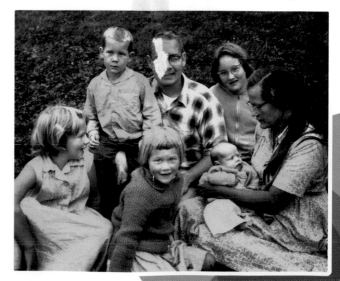

Still, it was painful to make room in the family for the prodigal father. Dotti, who had managed years of single parenting, now had to reaccept a husband who doubted his faith and himself, and depended on her support. It took years for Bill to get back on solid ground spiritually and emotionally, and more years for his children to once again respect and love their father. That it was even possible says volumes about Dotti's profound faith and her willingness to forgive.

> **"Think with your heart, not with your head."**
> *Dotti*

Although her personality was strong, Dotti's health was fragile. Since young adulthood, she'd borne up under countless infirmities resulting in numerous hospitalizations. The arthritis Dotti had been diagnosed with in her teens finally slowed her down in her sixties. Two painful knee replacements were immediately followed by a freak accident in a parking lot, when a car ran over Dotti's foot, crushing her ankle. Reconstructive surgery with lots of hardware followed. After some healing, the metal screws and plates were surgically removed. Dotti proudly displayed them in an empty peanut butter jar on a window sill in her living room. Following the accident, Dotti never really recovered the ability to walk any distance and often had to submit to being pushed in a wheelchair, or to using her preferred mode of mobility – her camo-painted scooter.

Decades of unrelenting pain have a way of making one intolerant of small talk or social niceties. Never one to engage in trivialities, Dotti became downright intense and would deliver shocking one-liners to those who she felt needed a jolt to inwardly wake up. One young father got a lesson in parenting when Dotti brought him up short by yelling, "Say it like you mean it when you call your children in from play. Otherwise they'll know you don't expect them to obey!"

Like Dorothy Day, whom she admired, Dotti's social radicalism was combined with a solidly orthodox faith. She had a "take no prisoners" approach to what she knew was true, and yet she retained an irrepressible love for all people and a desire for every one of them to find God. Her last job in the community was self-appointed. She loved to work over the stiff English translations of German sermons to make them interesting and understandable by "high school boys" – her favorite audience.

Dotti could smell a fake a mile away. She would have nothing to do with an empty, pious, or hypocritical religion. For Dotti, there was only one thing worse than politics and politicians – religious hypocrites. Her obvious love of Jesus and of the community confirmed my own decision to give myself to the same calling: to commit to a life holding all things in common, a life in full Christian community.

Ellen made a farewell visit to her

parents in Brooklyn to tell them she was now a Christian – and that her new faith was calling her to move to what in their eyes was a highly dubious commune off in England. ("What did we do wrong?" her father asked.) Then she returned to Wheathill, where after two years she married Ulrich Keiderling, a German craftsman. Together they had seven children. Then came 1977, a year that the family would

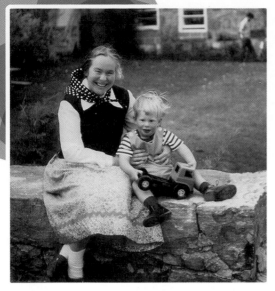

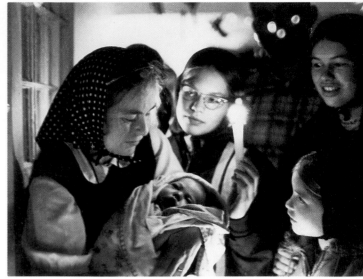

Ellen with Marie Johanna

always remember as a crucible of suffering and redemption. In February, three-year-old Mark John, the youngest and the apple of his parents' eye, was diagnosed with a rare, aggressive brain cancer. His parents and six older siblings spent the next three months caring for Mark John, preparing him for his inevitable death. They spared no effort to comfort him as he wasted away, became blind, and finally died in his parents' arms, fully trusting in Jesus to take him to heaven.

Just five months later, Ellen, now forty-five, went into labor with their eighth child. During delivery, Ellen was unconscious with no palpable pulse or blood pressure, taking both herself and her unborn daughter to the edge of death. During those hours, she experienced being irresistibly drawn toward the beauty of heaven. She always remembered smelling lilies and roses just before she was brought back to consciousness.

When Ellen awoke, though, she remembered little else. She did not recognize her own children, had no memory of Mark John's suffering and death, and did not know she had a new daughter. As she slowly regained her memory, she was forced to experience again the pain of losing Mark John and the dawning realization that she now needed to care for

another child who would not survive. Marie Johanna looked perfect, but was deemed "brain dead and incompatible with life." Throughout the two months she lived, she never opened her eyes and only cried twice. Ellen wrote:

> Marie Johanna's delicate, tender little body was with us, but her soul, right from the beginning, was stretched out between heaven and earth. We always thought of her as a messenger who would one day have to go back where she came from.

On Christmas Eve her children gathered around Ellen as she held Marie Johanna. One of her daughters held a candle next to the baby's face. Marie Johanna looked especially beautiful, Ellen remembered later. Then, for the first time, she opened her eyes. They were wide open and focused. She was looking into the corner of the room. At that moment, Ellen said:

> I felt our baby's soul leaving her. Her little soul rose from her body and passed in front of my face like a gentle, sweet breath. I was as certain of it as a blind person is sure when someone or something passes right by him. I felt wings brushing by my face – they were not soft, but stiff and strong, like the tips of birds' wings, but large – and with it a fragrance.

This is hard to put into words, but I felt this spiritual presence as surely as if it had been a physical presence. I stood transfixed for a moment, unable to move my head to look down at my baby. And when I did, what I saw only confirmed what I knew: her face was waxen, and she was no longer breathing.

Ellen had endured the most difficult experience a mother ever has to suffer – the death of a child. And she had been through it twice in less than a year. She later described that year as a time when "God had to shake us until our teeth rattled." But she and Ulrich let that unprecedented suffering soften and change them, and it guided the rest of their lives together. The change didn't happen overnight. Their children remember what felt like a long, dark time: days that turned into weeks when Ellen would retreat to her darkened bedroom to grieve and was not to be disturbed, years when Ulrich was away from the family working through his pain and finding his way back though his own inner wilderness.

"Where your treasure is," we are told, "There your heart will be also" (Matt. 6:21). Her children had gone ahead of her to the kingdom of heaven, and, as Ellen offered her pain to God, she found that she was able to cry out with great fervor for this kingdom to come. After 1977, Ellen refused novocaine at the dentist, celebrated being outside in cold weather, and embraced other discomforts in solidarity with her little boy who had gone through such pain. She emerged from that season of suffering as almost a new person.

The old originality was still there, now unleashed and deepened, setting her free to say and do whatever her heart said was true and right. Ulrich was back at her side, constant in his quiet love, cheering her on, occasionally reining in her excesses, and wordlessly giving her permission to speak from that place of pain and joy they'd gone through together.

That's the Ellen I met twenty years later. There was nothing grim about her. Like Elizabeth Bennet in Jane Austen's *Pride and Prejudice,* she dearly loved to laugh – at the absurdities of daily life, at a story by James Thurber, often at herself. She was exuberant in her love for individual people, for humanity, and for the church community that had carried her through those dark years. As Ellen once expressed:

> That's why each one of us is here, because we feel that here we can most closely and nearly live for that kingdom and give our lives for it, because we long for God's kingdom to come to the world. And we have this wonderful and precious task: that we can live for it and witness to it in every aspect of our lives, in every relationship – between husband and wife and between parents and children and brothers and sisters.

Doris knew pain of a different kind. Her suffering was like a long slow burn, kept below the surface where no one could see it. The love of her husband, Bud, a warm, outgoing, and energetic man, reassured her through the constant thoughts of self-doubt and self-accusation that sought to paralyze her spirit. In a low moment some years after joining the community, Doris questioned her motivations for doing so in the first place. She worried that

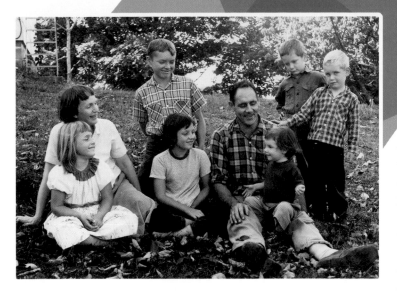

her decision had been based on her own principles, not on a loving response to a call. "I felt I was holding the lantern," she would later say, "but the lantern had no flame in it. Jesus was an ideal, but he was not my personal friend." Living on an ideal can work for a while – it sustained Bud and Doris for ten active years in the community – but then they felt the need to retreat with their family to rediscover Jesus himself.

During those years away from the community, Doris's feelings of inadequacy fueled her struggle to find a personal faith. She didn't want to just go through the motions of a committed life, but wanted her commitment to be real. She worried about inauthenticity; at times, her desire to live a genuine faith made it impossible for her to read the Bible to herself or her children without feeling hypocritical. She later wrote:

> Repentance was a mystery to me – something I knew I should have – but what was it?
>
> I had to face guilt and shame and hardly knew how, until one evening, listening to [Handel's] *Messiah*, I heard the words "The kingdom of this world is become the kingdom of our God." I suddenly was aware of the meaning of these words for me personally.

After this, slowly courage came and humility, and reconciliation began to take place. Repentance crept in quietly, without being named or recognized.

This was a beginning, the finding of a key, but for years still I struggled to find something that Bud had found. He could sit and read the Bible or other inner books, and be warmed and refreshed by it as though he were sitting by a warm fire.

Bud and Doris returned to the community in 1976, and spent ten golden years as youth counselors. Toward the end of that decade, Doris had a presentiment that she might not have many more years with Bud. A few months later, in June of 1986, she had to face her greatest fear when Bud was diagnosed with cancer. He died in December.

Doris spent the next thirty years as a widow. Whenever she felt lonely, she would sit at her desk and think of someone who might also be lonely and write them a letter. She wrote thousands of letters over those three decades, at least one a day and often more on the weekends. She corresponded with several inmates, many of whom wrote to the family after she died expressing their thankfulness for her faithful correspondence. Here's how Doris saw her ministry of writing in her later years:

> "Repentance was a mystery to me – something I knew I should have – but what was it?"
> *Doris*

Doris's artwork

Dotti, 2016 →

There are many ways of thinking of writing a letter. You can just sit down and start writing until you feel that you are done – or you can think about what gives Life meaning at the moment. It's a little bit like being born again for a third time!

Radiance

Because I'd met them separately and in their later years, it never occurred to me that these three women had much in common. Then they died one after the other, one month apart. And so, once a month for three months, I sat at each one's funeral and listened to their stories. That's when I saw the shape of what they shared beyond their membership in the same community. I realized each of them had discovered the value in something that so many of us work so hard to avoid – suffering.

What did all that suffering do for them? It wounded them. And living with their wounds made them both vulnerable and compassionate, and yet also bluntly honest. All that pain revealed to them that they were not in control of their lives, and never had been. It refined them like a blowtorch burns the dross off molten silver in a crucible, purifying the metal until it shines, indicating it is ready to be poured into a mold. Their crucible of suffering purified their intentions, leaving them with no option but to act and speak from their hearts. They each emerged from it with a depth of joy and freedom that drew me to them.

In her later years, one of Ellen's favorite things to do was to host an evening of poetry. She asked everyone to bring a poem or piece of inspiring prose to read aloud at the gathering. Before the reading started, Ellen made sure we were all comfortable – that is, that we had enough wine. And as the evening went on she kept the refills coming. Those gatherings held such good memories that her children hosted a beautiful poetry and prose evening – with wine, of course – the night before her funeral. As I sat there listening to her favorite poems being read, and her favorite sweet-sad songs being played by her grandson on his violin, I realized, "This is one measure of a life well lived." The most remarkable thing about Ellen's life was Ellen herself, but her radiance was not the result of her own efforts or achievements or decisions. It was Jesus, his suffering and resurrection, shining through her like light through stained glass.

Doris was granted her own kind of radiance. At an early age she had set her face toward the good and ruthlessly opposed any hint of selfishness in her own heart. For decades, her suffering, her dark night of the soul, was that she didn't always have the assurance that she was in God's presence; she craved it, perceiving what seemed like his absence in the face of evil.

The reality of God was so important to her that she did not want to fake a relationship she felt she had never experienced. She didn't doubt, but she longed for inner reassurance from God. Why is it that God sometimes hides his face from those who most faithfully follow and long for him? Doris's aridity reminds me of that of Mother Teresa, another woman

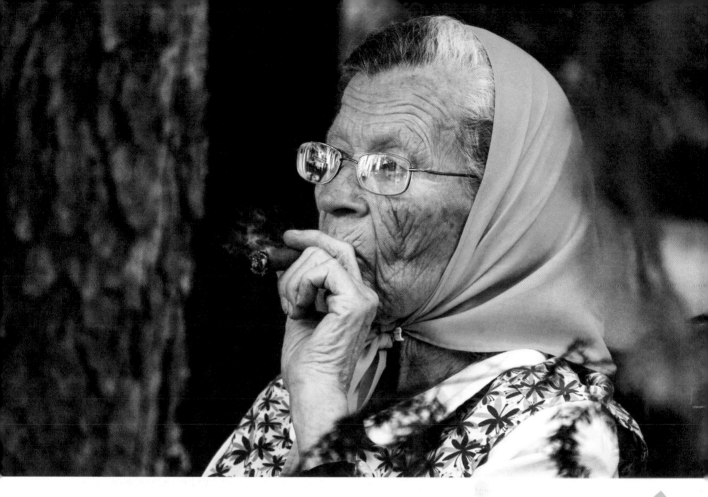

who experienced years of following what she knew was true without the interior affirmation of his close presence. Like the saint from Calcutta, Doris suffered under this perceived absence – yet continued in faith, undeterred and outwardly calm.

With Dotti, of course, life was never calm for long. She faced her wounds by speaking out, breaking the mold of what nice elderly women did and did not do, say, or wear. There's no denying she did it to get attention, but that attention was not for herself; with her bright colors she was like a flag, alerting people to the God in whom she was rooted. He was far more true and real than anything else she'd experienced in this world.

Dotti's health declined throughout the ten months after Bill died. She'd stopped eating numerous times only to restart, and was completely wheelchair bound. Yet two weeks before she died she made one final splash when she was wheeled into a community celebration. Her favorite Louis Armstrong song was playing: "What a Wonderful World." Dotti somehow got out of her chair, and started to dance. It began as a shuffle but then her crippled feet caught the music and moved into the old-time box step. She grinned from ear to ear as one young man after another took her hands and followed her lead. After a full ten minutes of dancing, she was helped back into her wheelchair, exhausted but triumphant – as if certain that her life had been well lived.

"God had to shake us until our teeth rattled."
Ellen

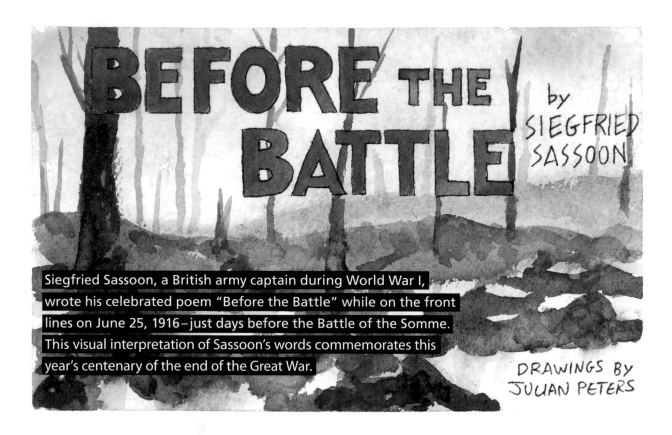

BEFORE THE BATTLE
by SIEGFRIED SASSOON

Siegfried Sassoon, a British army captain during World War I, wrote his celebrated poem "Before the Battle" while on the front lines on June 25, 1916–just days before the Battle of the Somme. This visual interpretation of Sassoon's words commemorates this year's centenary of the end of the Great War.

DRAWINGS BY JULIAN PETERS

MUSIC OF WHISPERING TREES

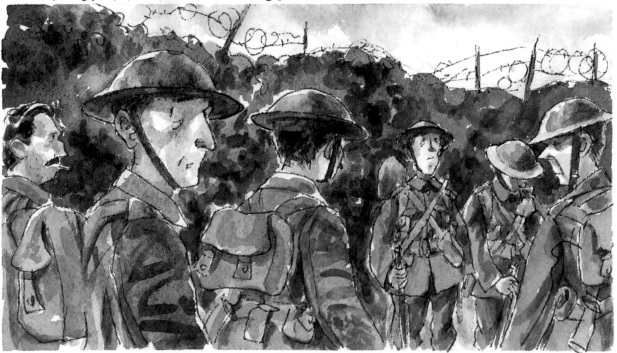

HUSHED BY A BROAD-WINGED BREEZE

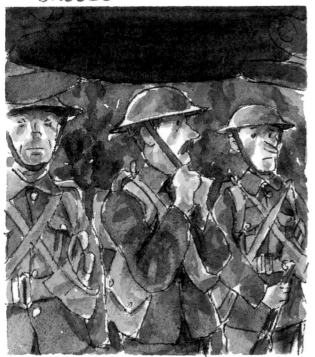

WHERE SHAKEN WATER GLEAMS;

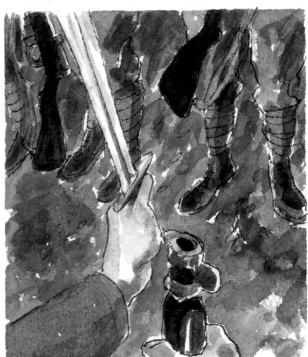

AND EVENING RADIANCE FALLING

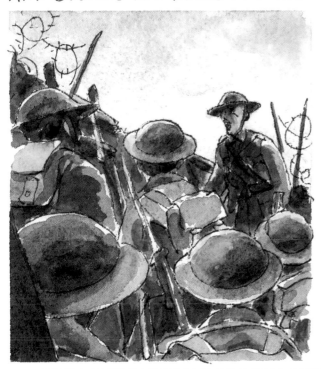

WITH REEDY BIRD-NOTES CALLING.

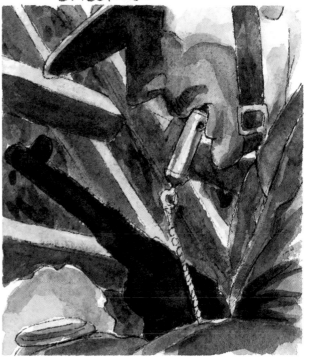

Julian Peters is an illustrator and comic book artist living in Montreal, Canada, who focuses on adapting classical poems into graphic art. julianpeterscomics.com

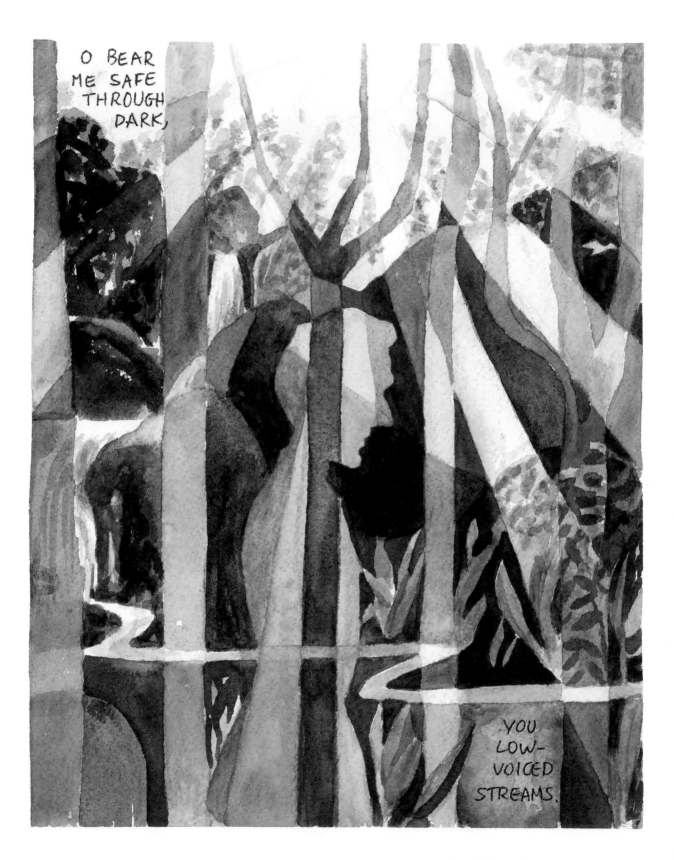

I HAVE NO NEED TO PRAY

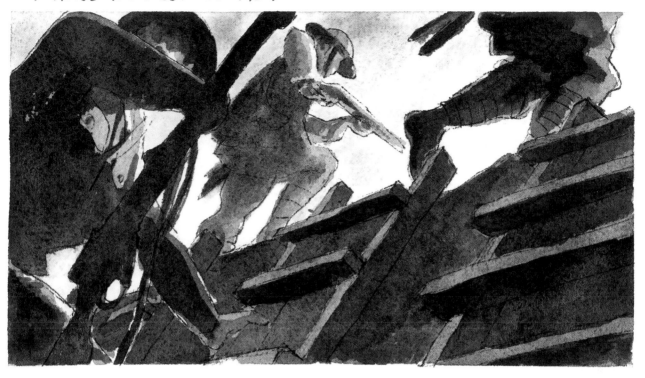

THAT FEAR MAY PASS AWAY;

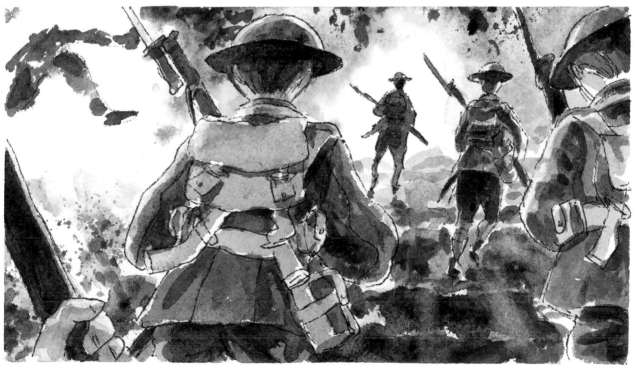

I SCORN THE GROWL AND RUMBLE OF THE FIGHT

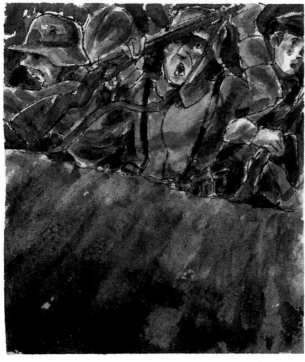

THAT SUMMONS ME FROM COOL

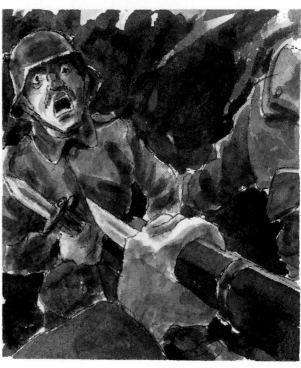

SILENCE OF MARSH AND POOL

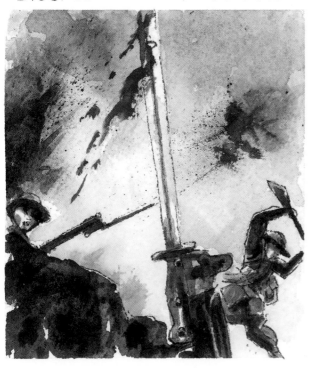

AND YELLOW LILIES ISLANDED IN LIGHT

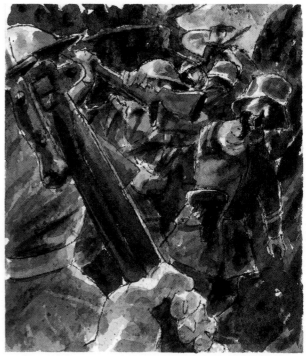

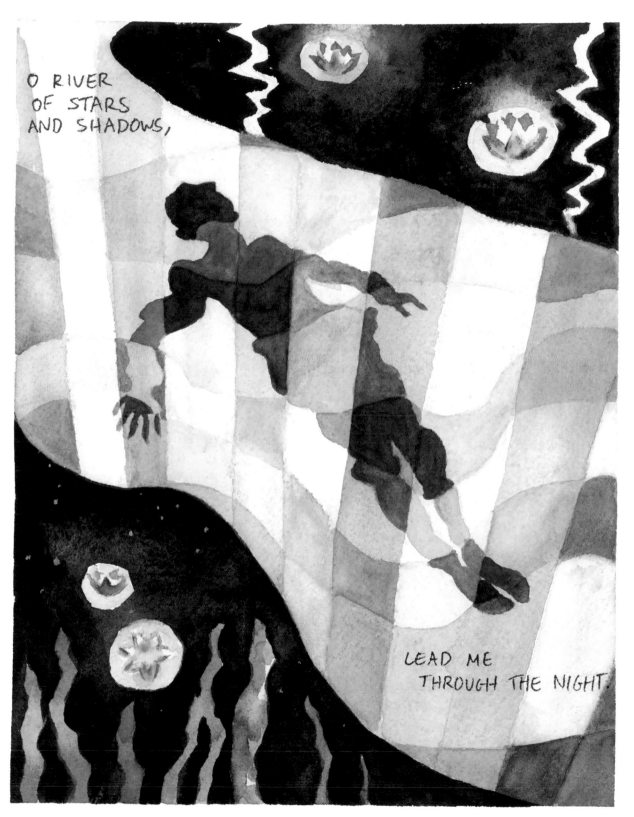

THE END

Editors' Picks

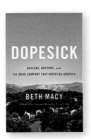

Dopesick: Dealers, Doctors, and the Drug Company that Addicted America
Beth Macy
(Little, Brown)

In *Dopesick,* journalist Beth Macy gives the opioid epidemic a human face, but not at the expense of historical and scientific context. This epidemic, she argues, can be traced to the greed of one pharmaceutical company. Purdue Pharma's release of OxyContin in 1996 led to an epidemic of iatrogenic (doctor-caused) opioid addiction, the third in US history. The first epidemic had led to the deaths of countless Civil War veterans to morphine; the second had killed off thousands of middle-class housewives before heroin was banned in 1924, twenty-six years after its release as an over-the-counter drug. But Purdue couldn't have succeeded without thousands of unscrupulous doctors and sales reps who cashed in at the expense of the most susceptible. OxyContin's arrival also coincided with patients becoming healthcare consumers and pain becoming "the fifth vital sign," to be avoided at all costs. Not treating pain was tantamount to abuse, preached the new medical experts funded by Big Pharma. It wasn't long before courts and prisons were overwhelmed as addicts started stealing from their families and neighbors and switching to heroin, not seeking a high but simply to stave off the "dopesickness" of withdrawal.

Treatment, regulation, education, and new criminal justice approaches are all urgently needed, but it will take more than that to stem the great tide of despair of which this scourge is but a symptom.

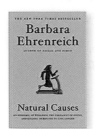

Natural Causes: An Epidemic of Wellness, the Certainty of Dying, and Killing Ourselves to Live Longer
Barbara Ehrenreich
(Twelve)

Our bodies don't always function as a harmonious whole. Macrophages, those good cells in our immune system that eat pathogens, also aid and abet the spread of cancer and have been implicated in arthritis, Alzheimer's, and diabetes. "The fire department is indeed staffed by arsonists," writes Barbara Ehrenreich (*Nickel and Dimed*). So, despite our efforts, we're going to die.

At 76, Ehrenreich knows she's old enough to die of "natural causes" – and she isn't about to waste her remaining years denying herself butter and wine or subjecting herself to invasive medical treatment to stave off the inevitable. With wit and verve, she takes aim at excessive cancer screening, the medicalization of childbearing, the fitness and wellness industries, fad diets, faux-Buddhist mindfulness, self-help gurus, and much more. Medical professionals may find some of her generalizations unfair, but her main indictment is reserved for us, consumers in a culture obsessed with self.

The self has supplanted God as the object of our worship and replaced the soul as the essence of our being. An atheist herself, Ehrenreich senses that it's a sorry substitute, but fails to offer a way out. For her, it's enough to die in a world seething with life, knowing the blackbirds will go on singing without her. As consolation many will find this rather thin, and Ehrenreich's solutions likewise are hardly satisfying (unless you count psychedelic drugs that temporarily suppress the selfish zone of your brain). Yet Ehrenreich is an acute diagnostician of our society's pathologies, and her book is as serious as it is entertaining.

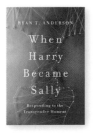

When Harry Became Sally: Responding to the Transgender Moment
Ryan T. Anderson
(Encounter)

In this book, Ryan T. Anderson explores the arguments at the heart of the growing confusion about gender identity and sexuality. Acknowledging the real psychological suffering that people with gender dysphoria experience, he describes how that suffering can be increased by mistaken medical treatment, and addresses the social changes that gender-theory activists are demanding.

To Anderson, there are basic contradictions in the beliefs that these activists promote. They believe that the real self is fundamentally separate from the body – that it's possible for a boy to "really" be a girl – yet at the same time they insist that the body matters after all, since it's crucial to medically transform it to match one's felt identity. Similarly, activists tie authentic gender identity to stereotypically male and female activities while also claiming that gender is an artificial and fluid construct. What's more, this artificial construct trumps the biological realities that humans have always taken as markers of male and female. As a result, those struggling with their gender identity may be prescribed radical and invasive "therapies": puberty blockers, cross-sex hormones, and surgeries.

Anderson calls for compassion for those who suffer from gender confusion. At the same time, he points out that sex is inscribed into our bodies, down to the DNA in every cell.

Being male or female is thus not something we can choose or change; surgery cannot replace chromosomes. Sex, Anderson writes, "is a bodily, biological reality, and gender is how we give social expression to that reality. Gender properly understood is a social manifestation of human nature, springing forth from biological realities, though shaped by rational and moral choice." Our bodies are part of who we are, not something external to ourselves in which we find our real selves trapped.

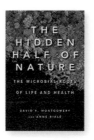

The Hidden Half of Nature: The Microbial Roots of Life and Health
David R. Montgomery and Anne Biklé
(W. W. Norton)

Geologist David R. Montgomery and his wife, Anne Biklé, a biologist, collaborate in this fascinating book to reveal the uncanny parallels between healthy soil and healthy bodies. Couched as a memoir, it records their personal journey rehabilitating a chemically devastated lawn into a thriving vegetable garden while Anne recovers from cancer. Research continues to expose the role of the "hidden half of nature," the microbial world that sustains life on our planet, in the soil and in our bodies, which are not just us but also a complex community of microbes we host – their cells outnumber ours at least three to one. Eighty percent of our immune system is the work of these guests in our intestine and colon, where over a thousand unique species live and work for us. An awareness of these dependencies is game-changing, as we come to realize that so much of what we commonly do is deadly to what maintains life; not only pesticides and herbicides but also sanitizers, food processing, and antibiotics need a closer look. We have a lot to learn, and here are two enthusiastic teachers. ➤ *The Editors*

The Beguines

JASON LANDSEL

"Men try to dissuade me from everything Love bids me do. They don't understand it, and I can't explain it to them. I must live out what I am," wrote Hadewijch, a thirteenth-century woman from Antwerp, Belgium.

Hadewijch was a member of the Beguines, a medieval renewal movement of women – there was a brother movement for men known as the Beghards – that formed around 1200 in Flanders and lasted until 2013, when Marcella Pattyn, the last Beguine, died.

The Beguines were lay women who formed communities of worship and mutual economic support. While some beguinages were loosely aligned with religious orders, they remained independent from the hierarchical and financial structures of Europe's medieval church. While renowned for their zeal in prayer and their charitable works, which made them indispensable in many towns, the Beguines were often under suspicion. Several were pronounced heretics, and even executed, for their mystical teachings or for "insubordination."

Nevertheless, the movement grew. Drawn by new employment opportunities in growing industries, many women came to cities for employment. There, cut off from the traditional social network of extended families and tight-knit rural villages, they turned to beguinages for support and fellowship. Others, drawn to a life of apostolic service, came from upper-class backgrounds. Some were widows or fleeing abusive marriages; still others were rescued from a life of begging or prostitution.

The Beguines practiced a simple lifestyle, but still owned property individually and communally. Members were free to leave the community at any time. Beguinages differed in size, from a single house with a few women to a walled village with over a thousand inhabitants. Communities were frequently guided by a *magistra,* a woman of eloquence and spiritual insight.

Beguines were committed to *vita apostolica* – the "apostolic life." French historian Jaques de Vitry described beguinages as "hospices of piety, houses of honesty, workshops of holiness, convents of the right and devout life, refuges of the poor, sustenance to the wretched, consolation to those in mourning, refectories for the hungry, comfort and relief for those who are ill." Beyond these acts of mercy, the Beguines carried out an energetic street ministry, with plays and theaters that urged audiences to repent and turn back to the source of their faith.

The movement produced numerous visionaries and mystics – women like Marguerite Porete, Mechtild of Magdeburg, and Hadewijch – whose visions, prayers, poems, and spiritual practices were documented and survive as inspiration to this day. ⟶

"Love is always new! Those who live in Love are renewed every day and through their frequent acts of goodness are born all over again. How can anyone stay old in Love's presence? How can anyone be timid there?"

Hadewijch

Jason Landsel is the artist for Plough's *"Forerunners" series, including the painting opposite, after Rogier van der Weyden's* Portrait of a Young Woman *(c. 1435).*